There's Always More

A JOURNEY TO SELF-DISCOVERY

GO BEYOND ME
BOOK THREE

SUSAN STIVER

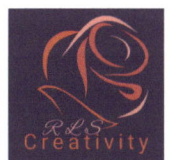

Foreword

I'm thanking You, God,
from a full heart,
I'm writing the book
on Your wonders.
Psalm 9:1 (The Message)

There's more to life than just a career –
It's the relationships all along the way,
And discovering the depths of
who you are,
and who you were created to be.

This book is dedicated

First to my parents who let me be me,
and to Don who encouraged me
to be who God created me to be.

Then to nurses everywhere,
But especially to those from
Johnston-Willis Hospital
School of Nursing,
And
To all of the men and women with whom I have had
the privilege of working side by side in hospitals
for over four decades of my life.

And last, but not least,
To all those who will be brave enough
To begin their own journey
To self-discovery!

Acknowledgments

I thank God for the career He handpicked for me,
And for His hand that led me
through all those years.

Special thanks to Martha Gregory,
who first invited me into the medical field
as a Junior Volunteer,
and
to Dr. Onufer who opened the door
of the NICU to me.

Extra special thanks to Diane Johnson,
who set an example, and encouraged me
to strive for nursing excellence.

Deep heartfelt gratitude to
Jeannene Whitefield Mitchell,
Who was the first person in my life
Telling me to publish my poetry.
She saw the creative part of me -
That's what dear friends do.

Contents

Preface

In the grand scheme of life, as crazy and chaotic as it can be, have you ever wondered who you are, or what makes *you* be you? Or pondered about your purpose or worth? Is there some extravagant, out-of-reach master plan eluding us that has not yet been revealed? Most people are too young, or too busy to stop and consider these queries. I believe that we are all individuals created by the meticulous design of a Master Craftsman. There are no cookie-cutter people. No two are alike! That is part of what makes life, real life, so exciting and enjoyable.

My initial plan for this book was to loosely write memoirs about my career as a nurse, but it became so much more. While looking through keepsakes that my mother had saved over the years, to my surprise –
I found ME.

It's my hope that you will slow down just long enough to have your curiosity piqued, and take this challenge to embark on your own journey to self-discovery. You won't regret it.

Nursing Career
NOT BY CHOICE, BUT CHOSEN!

The Medical World is a complex maze of offices, physicians, nurses, clients, diagnoses, treatments, policies, procedures, ups, and downs – not a career choice I would have considered as a teenager in my ninth grade
Civics class.
At least not until...
My best friend Martha invited me to join her as a Junior Volunteer at a local Hospital. From that moment on, my life was forever changed.
I had discovered my purpose, and being in the Hospital environment came as natural to me as breathing.
I was in my element, and I realized that I was created for this calling. God designed me for bedside care, and equipped me to be a patient advocate.

He poured into me the skill set and knowledge I would need to provide critical care for the most vulnerable patient population - preterm and sick newborn infants. To my skill set He added an extra measure of critical thinking, problem solving, and compassion.
My head and my heart were full.

Over the years it was always an honor and privilege to care
for these little ones.
It was great joy to help the parents grow into,
and assume their role as the care giver.

As with all positions and life situations, there were challenges to be faced and addressed, struggles to overcome, obstacles to work around, but in the end, the reward made it all worthwhile. Worthwhile enough to go back to do it again and again and again...day after day after day for forty-one years.
I will be forever grateful to God for the career He handpicked for me, and for His hand that guided me through all those years.

The Nevers

In the course of your life, have you ever said you'd **never** do something? And how did that work for you?

Early on in life I had some pretty definite "**nevers**". Happy to be in my family, one day I announced that I would **never** get married, and I would **never** have children. Up until my ninth-grade civics class, I was sure I would **never** be a nurse. Well, after the first chapter you already know how that turned out. Having been a junior volunteer in the hospital, I had added to my list of "**nevers**". I would **never** work in OB (Obstetrics). However, while in training, I learned that OB wasn't really bad, but I would **never** work in the nursery, and certainly **never** with sick babies. During that phase of my training, we had to work night shift with premature infants. That became my life's breath. To top it off, night shift and I were a perfect fit! By this time, most of my "**nevers**" were crossed off the list that I had so adamantly proclaimed. Then in the second year of nursing school I got married. Seems that everything I had said I would **never** do was being required of me. God was working on His plan for my life. That last "**never**" of having no children? That, too, was canceled seven years later. All part of God's perfect plan.

Where It All Began

Would you believe this all started when I was born??? Sounds strange, and I almost didn't believe it either until... looking back to being born in the wee hours of one cold December night, and being told stories of staying up all night until my father's alarm clock went off for him to get up, then I would go to sleep... Just sayin'.

As a youngster, I was a typical middle child busy getting into my older sister's stuff, and fussing with my younger siblings. I think I remember something that says middle children are the reason families have to make rules. Not a bad kid – just needed some boundaries. Then I followed those guidelines fairly closely, because I didn't like being in trouble.

Oops! That just brought back an early childhood memory. Kindergarten. Being totally honest, I was the teacher's biggest challenge that year. One rainy day, I remember carrying my umbrella to my desk with me. The teacher tried to reason with me, "Susan, all of the other children have put their umbrellas in the closet." When I didn't budge, she took my umbrella. Without saying a word, I got up, went to the closet, put on my raincoat, and wore it all day. Well, you know what that meant – a trip to the principal's office. Dare I say, that was not the first, nor the last time, I visited Ms. Dewey in her office. It's pretty bad that I can so quickly recall her name, but had to find my old report card to realize my kindergarten teacher even had a name. My nearly perfect attendance that year was no consolation to her, and of course, she would recommend that I be promoted to the next grade. But on that very same report card, she left one word for me to discover – "Creative." She wrote the word "Creative"! WOW! She saw into me! Reviewing some of the other report cards my mother had in her keepsakes – there it was. "Outstandings" and "A's" in all my writing and art classes. I had never put 2 and 2 together until now. Truthfully, this realization has only recently come to me as I have been retrospectively reviewing my life, to explore and discover what made me be me. That creative part of me went dormant for years — overridden by a life twist I experienced in the ninth grade.

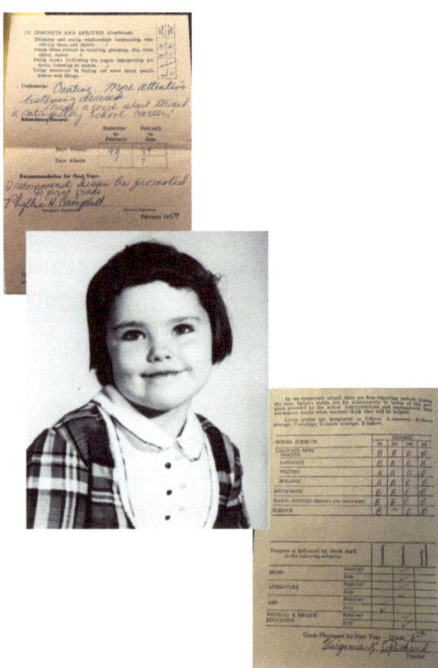

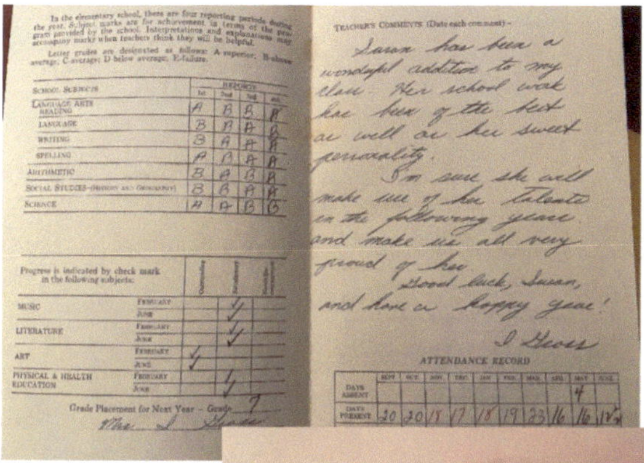

In the elementary school, there are four reporting periods during the year. Subject marks are for achievement in terms of the program provided by the school. Interpretations and explanations may accompany marks when teachers think they will be helpful.

Letter grades are designated as follows: A-superior; B-above average; C-average; D-below average; E-failure.

School Subjects	Reports 1st	2nd	3rd	4th
Language Arts Reading	A	B	B	A
Language	B	A	A	B
Writing	B	A	A	A
Spelling	A	A	A	A
Arithmetic	B	A	B	A
Social Studies—(History and Geography)	B	B	A	A
Science	A	A	B	B

Progress is indicated by check mark in the following subjects:				
Music	February		✓	
	June		✓	
Literature	February		✓	
	June		✓	
Art	February	✓		
	June	✓		
Physical & Health Education	February		✓	
	June		✓	

Grade Placement for Next Year – Grade 7

Mrs. I. Gross

Teacher's Comments (Date each comment) –

Susan has been a wonderful addition to my class. Her school work has been of the best as well as her sweet personality.

I'm sure she will make use of her talents in the following years and make us all very proud of her.

Good luck, Susan, and have a happy year!

I. Gross

ATTENDANCE RECORD

	Sept	Oct	Nov	Dec	Jan	Feb	Mar	Apr	May	June
Days Absent									4	
Days Present	20	20	18	17	18	19	23	16	16	12

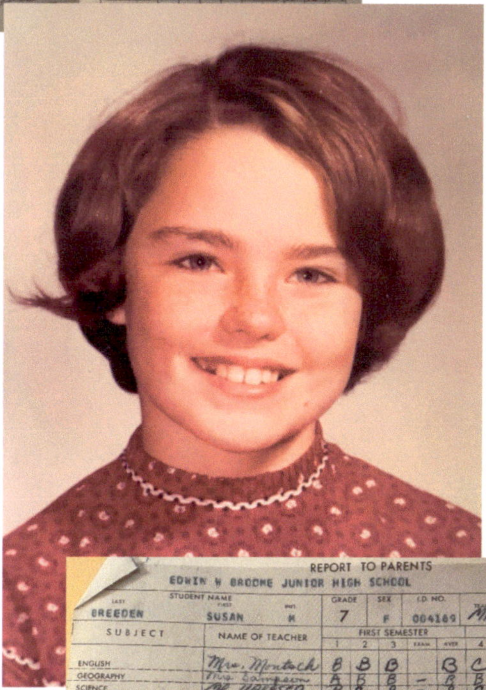

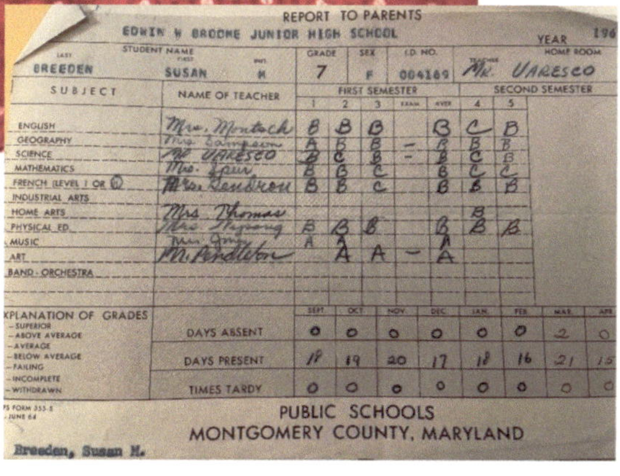

REPORT TO PARENTS

EDWIN W BROOME JUNIOR HIGH SCHOOL — YEAR 196

Student Name Last	First	Init.	Grade	Sex	I.D. No.	Home Room Teacher
BREEDEN	SUSAN	M	7	F	004169	Mr. Varesco

Subject	Name of Teacher	First Semester 1	2	3	Exam	Aver	Second Semester 4	5
English	Mrs. Montach	B	B	B		B	C	B
Geography	Mrs. Sampson	A	B	B	–	B	B	B
Science	Mr. Varesco	B	C	B	–	B	C	B
Mathematics	Mrs. Spur	B	B	C		B	C	C
French (Level I or II)	Mrs. Gendron	B	B	C		B	B	B
Industrial Arts								
Home Arts	Mrs Thomas						B	
Physical Ed	Mrs [illegible]	B	B	B		B	B	B
Music	Mrs. [illegible]	A	A			A		
Art	Mr. Pendleton		A	A	–	A		
Band - Orchestra								

Explanation of Grades
– Superior
– Above Average
– Average
– Below Average
– Failing
– Incomplete
– Withdrawn

	Sept	Oct	Nov	Dec	Jan	Feb	Mar	Apr
Days Absent	0	0	0	0	0	0	2	0
Days Present	18	19	20	17	18	16	21	15
Times Tardy	0	0	0	0	0	0	0	0

PS Form 355-5 – June 64

PUBLIC SCHOOLS
MONTGOMERY COUNTY, MARYLAND

Breeden, Susan M.

Ninth Grade Twist

With Elementary and Junior High School in the rear-view mirror – Hello High School! Somehow, I managed to stay under the radar for the most part, lost in the mass of students. Studying was hard for me. Oh, how I envied the audio learners. I might have been one of them, if I wasn't daydreaming in class. Then came the challenge – ninth grade civics class. The instructor gave us an assignment to explore career choices. All the girls chose Nursing. Seemed so redundant and boring to me. I was going to be different – maybe a little renegade-ish again. Psychiatry sounded more intriguing and lucrative. Our report was to include education requirements, length and cost of that education, all the way to the potential annual income. And what did I discover?

Becoming a Psychiatrist would require more years of education and expense than I had expected, or was willing to expend. My conclusion in the report was that I would most likely be the one on the couch instead of in the chair.

Then there was Martha. She was my best friend in the whole world. She was going to become a junior volunteer at the local hospital, and invited me to go with her. I figured I'd give it a try. This became the ninth-grade twist. From that moment on, my life was forever changed. There I discovered my purpose, and being in the Hospital environment became as natural to me as breathing.

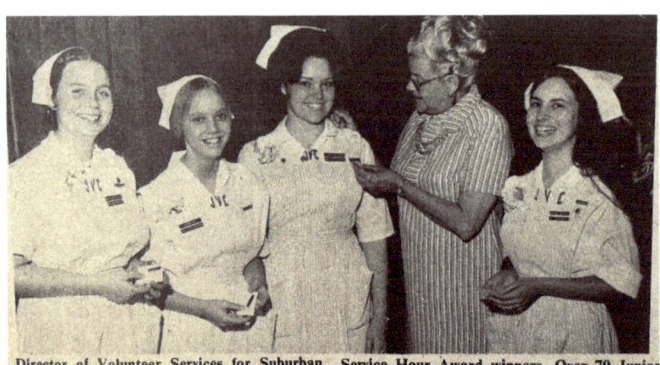

Director of Volunteer Services for Suburban Hospital, Mrs. Robert N. Crain, congratulates Junior Volunteers Hetty DeVroom, Donna Bolton, Sue Breeden and Donna Denny, all 400 Service Hour Award winners. Over 70 Junior Volunteers, representing eight area high schools, were honored recently at the hospital's Spring Awards Ceremony.

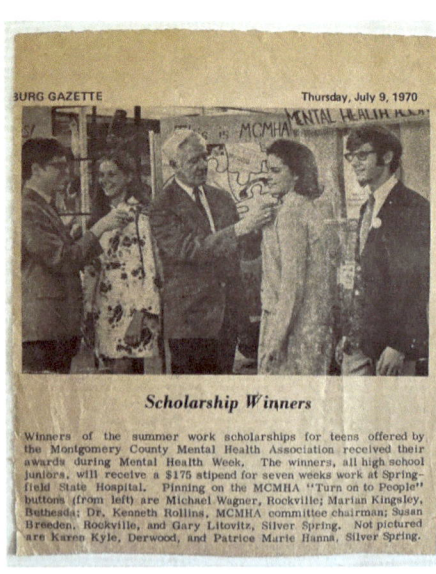

BURG GAZETTE   Thursday, July 9, 1970

Scholarship Winners

Winners of the summer work scholarships for teens offered by the Montgomery County Mental Health Association received their awards during Mental Health Week. The winners, all high school juniors, will receive a $175 stipend for seven weeks work at Springfield State Hospital. Pinning on the MCMHA "Turn on to People" buttons (from left) are Michael Wagner, Rockville; Marian Kingsley, Bethesda; Dr. Kenneth Rollins, MCMHA committee chairman; Susan Breeden, Rockville, and Gary Litovitz, Silver Spring. Not pictured are Karen Kyle, Derwood, and Patrice Marie Hanna, Silver Spring.

All of this is part of what made me be me. Instead of staying the kindergarten renegade, I became a Type A personality, who eventually went into Nursing - writing the policies and procedures for several hospitals, and articles on professional nursing practice and patient care, during my 41-year career. Not to mention I became a Night Shift Nurse by choice. God has a way of using everything in our lives to develop us into the individuals He created us to be.

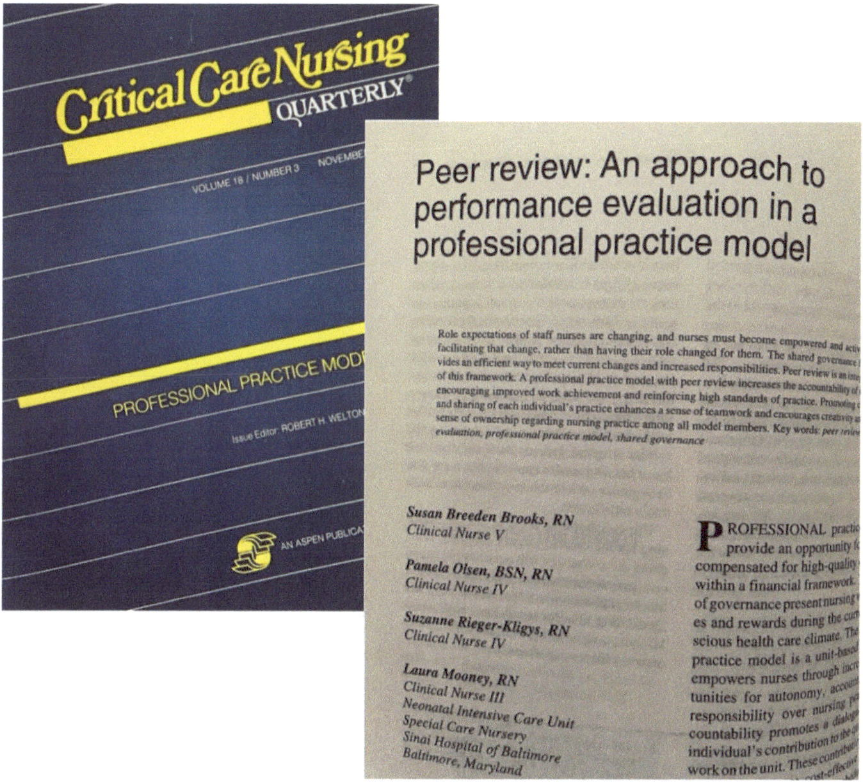

Critical Care Nursing QUARTERLY®

VOLUME 18 / NUMBER 3 NOVEMBE

PROFESSIONAL PRACTICE MODE

Issue Editor: ROBERT H. WELTON

AN ASPEN PUBLICA

Peer review: An approach to performance evaluation in a professional practice model

Role expectations of staff nurses are changing, and nurses must become empowered and active facilitating that change, rather than having their role changed for them. The shared governance vides an efficient way to meet current changes and increased responsibilities. Peer review is an in of this framework. A professional practice model with peer review increases the accountability of encouraging improved work achievement and reinforcing high standards of practice. Promoting and sharing of each individual's practice enhances a sense of teamwork and encourages creativity a sense of ownership regarding nursing practice among all model members. Key words: peer review evaluation, professional practice model, shared governance

Susan Breeden Brooks, RN
Clinical Nurse V

Pamela Olsen, BSN, RN
Clinical Nurse IV

Suzanne Rieger-Kligys, RN
Clinical Nurse IV

Laura Mooney, RN
Clinical Nurse III
Neonatal Intensive Care Unit
Special Care Nursery
Sinai Hospital of Baltimore
Baltimore, Maryland

P ROFESSIONAL practi
provide an opportunity f
compensated for high-quality
within a financial framework.
of governance present nursing
es and rewards during the cur
scious health care climate. The
practice model is a unit-bas
empowers nurses through incr
tunities for autonomy, accou
responsibility over nursing p
countability promotes a dialog
individual's contribution to the
work on the unit. These contrib

*Like an open book, you watched me grow from
conception to birth;
all the stages of my life were spread out before you,
The days of my life all prepared
before I'd even lived one day.
Psalm 139:16 (The Message)*

Rude Awakening

All my early life I thought I was living in the real world, until I went off to Nursing School. Reality hit me like a ton of bricks. Being the youngest student in a class of fifty was certainly a challenge. I might have been more comfortable had I been one of the middle children in the group. But now I was on my own, and four hours from home, with no escape. To help new students adjust to dorm life, and this altered reality, we were not allowed to have a car, or go home for a month. Thank goodness I was allowed to use the rotary dial phone to make calls to my parents, but the phone was in the main hall. We had to wait our turn to use the phone, and because there were so many of us wanting to use it, there was a time limit.

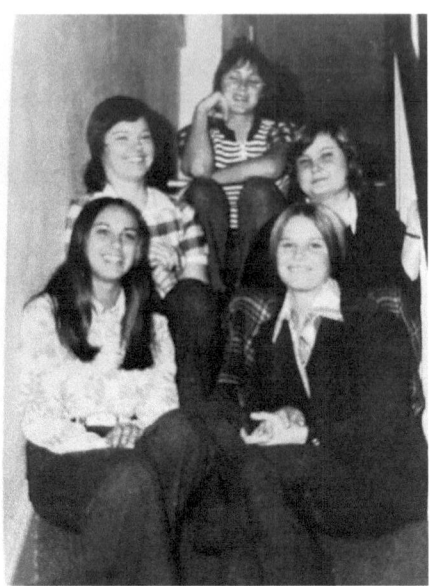

The staircase was a great place to wait for phone access, mail call, or visitors.

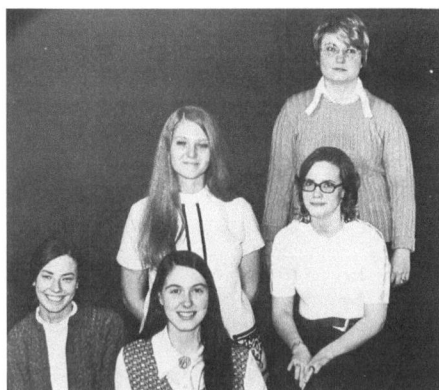

Dorm life was quite an adjustment! We had schedules for everything - classes, meals, floor duty, study hall, linen changes, curfews. The house mothers made sure we were where we were supposed to be, and when! Add to that - an extensive demerit system.

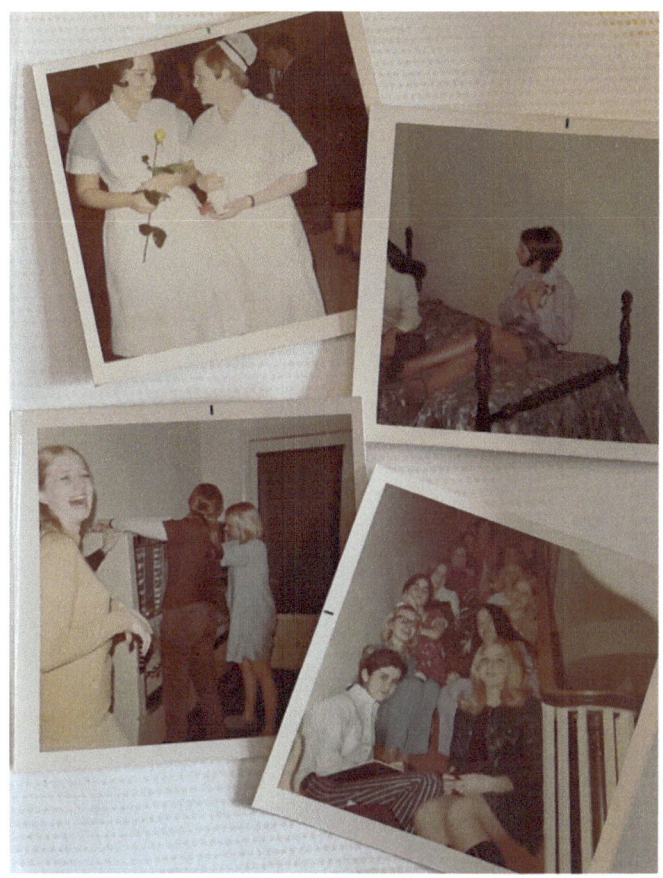

Each apartment was shared by an average of four girls. There was really no place to hide. So homesick that first month, I lost 18 pounds! It's actually a miracle I kept it off, as we eventually developed a habit of making trips to Aunt Sarah's Pancake House, and consuming quarts and half gallons of ice cream in the lounge during off hours. No bowls were required – just the spoons! Not to mention, desperately raiding the candy machines!

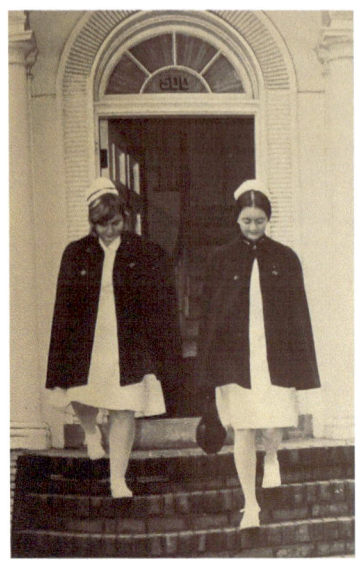

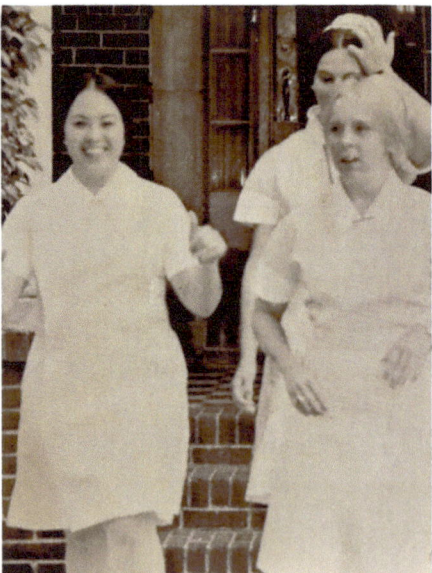

And for the first time in my life there was a strict dress code! Talk about rules and regulations. There were even rules about what we could and couldn't wear.

Total strangers quickly became forever friends.

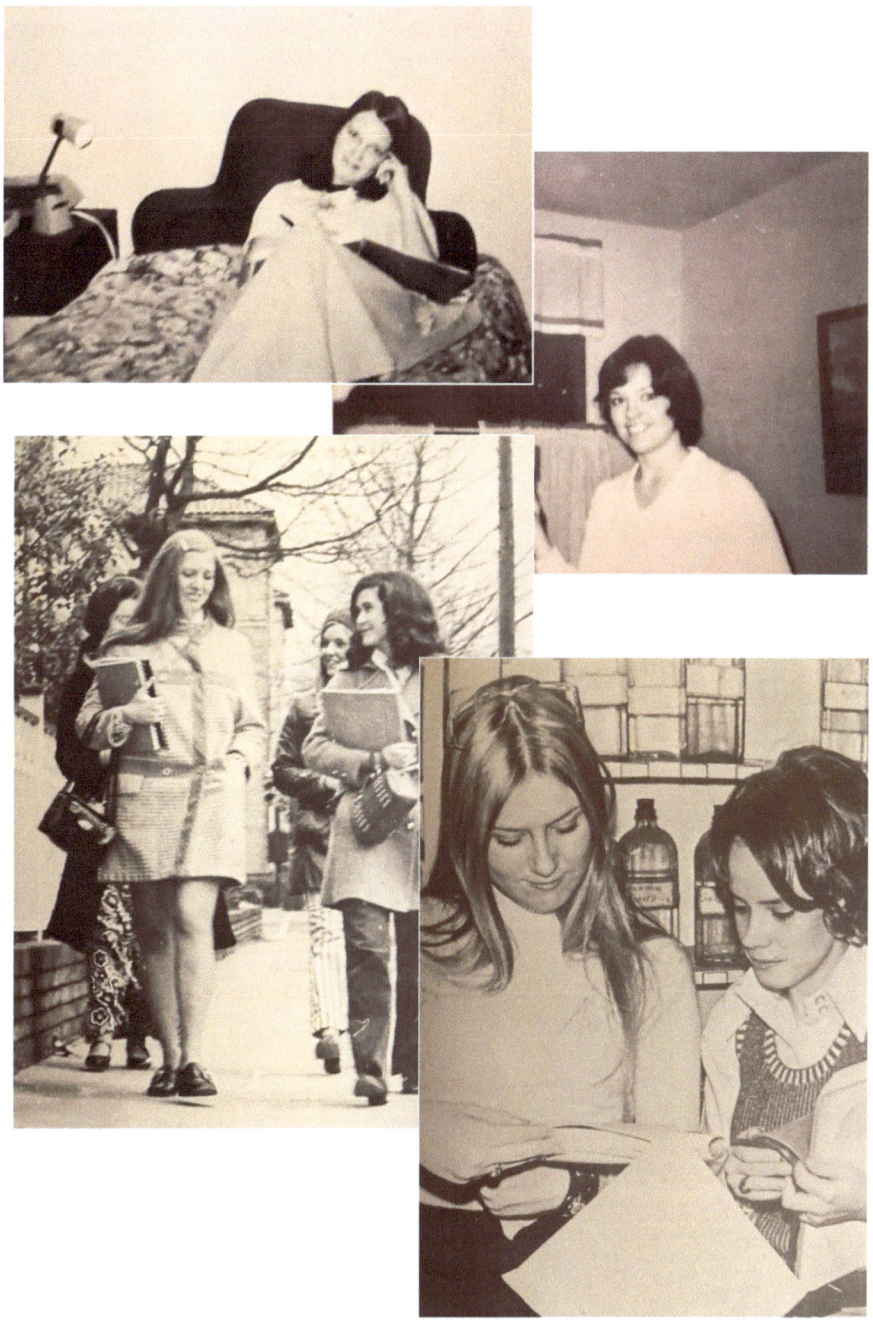

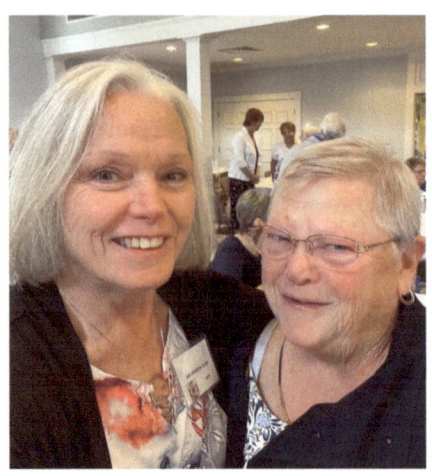

As scared as I was, I quickly learned that I was never alone. The school gave each of us a Big Sister from the senior class to help us transition to this new phase of life. Sharon just happened to be the best!

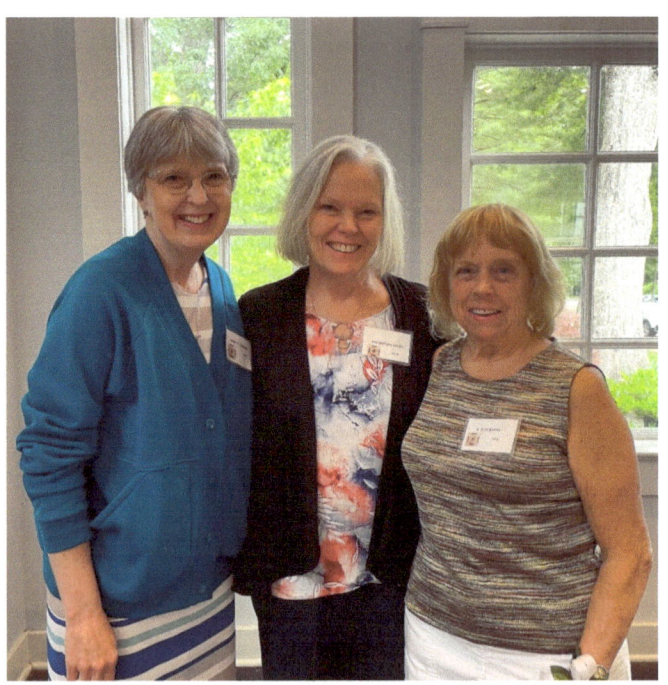

To that God kept adding more forever friends – Nancy, Jean, and a host of others.

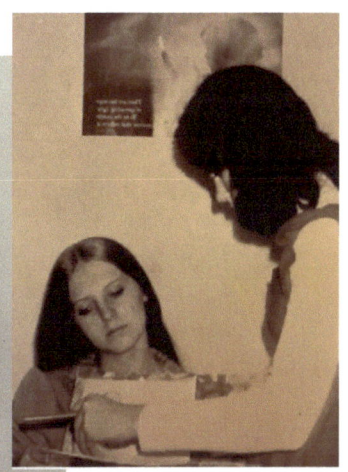

Everyday, in my encounters with others or in my studies, I find another part of myself. Each part helps to complete that which will one day be whole.

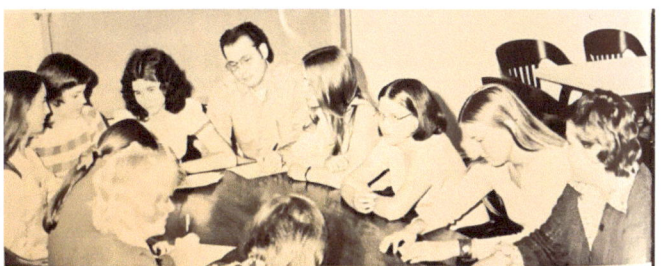

Nursing School was both challenging and rewarding. We studied long hours during the day, and pulled our share of night shifts as supplemental staff. It was exhilarating.

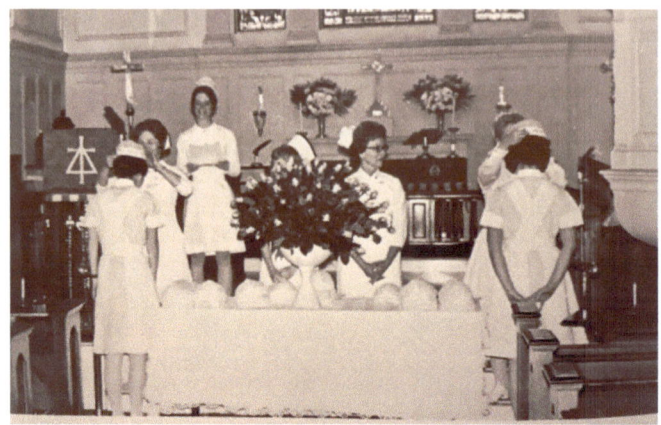

Over three years, we were not only taught the details of nursing, and entrusted with patient care, but we had also learned to respect each other as individuals, and professionals. We went from being kids to becoming responsible young adults.

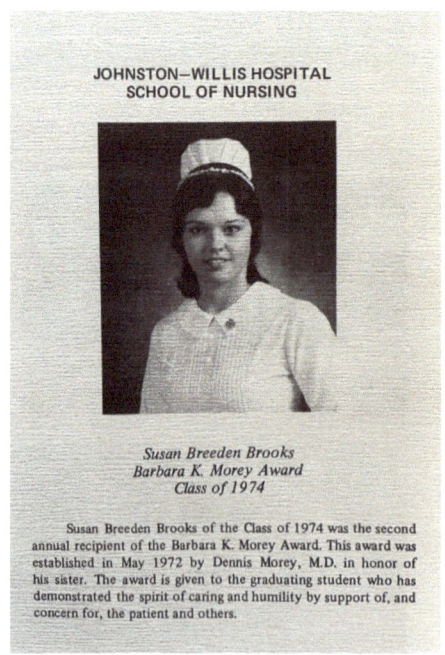

JOHNSTON–WILLIS HOSPITAL
SCHOOL OF NURSING

Susan Breeden Brooks
Barbara K. Morey Award
Class of 1974

Susan Breeden Brooks of the Class of 1974 was the second annual recipient of the Barbara K. Morey Award. This award was established in May 1972 by Dennis Morey, M.D. in honor of his sister. The award is given to the graduating student who has demonstrated the spirit of caring and humility by support of, and concern for, the patient and others.

To celebrate before graduation several of us went to the beach for a couple of days. Just let me say, it was quite uncomfortable wearing a long-sleeved starched uniform and panty hose over a blistered sunburn. Some of us had sunburnt faces that nearly matched the eighteen long stem red roses we carried during the ceremony that day. But we carried those roses with great satisfaction and pride!

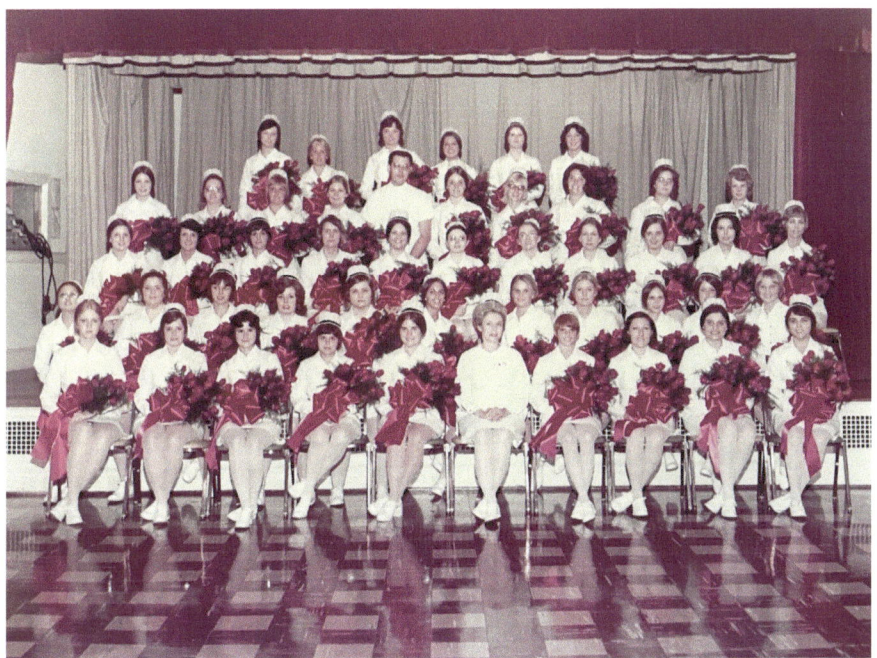

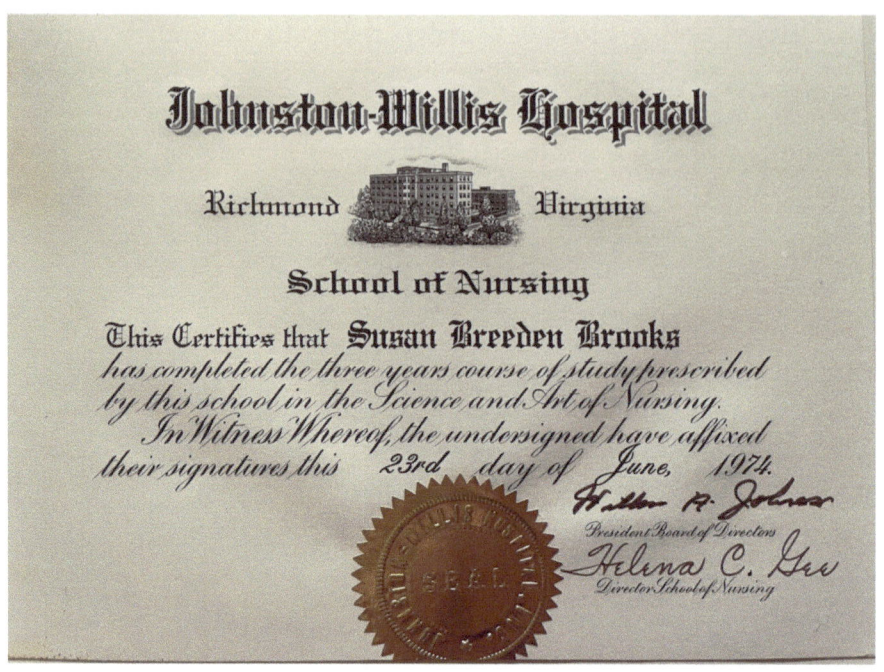

With this Certificate in hand,
it was now time to take the Nursing Boards, and step into my calling.

Pinch Me

Taking the Nursing Boards was a daunting two full-day ordeal. Oh, how we studied for this! The time came, then came the wait! Unlike the quick turnaround time with today's new technology, waiting for test results back then took weeks! I held my breath each time I went to the mailbox hoping that day would be the day I'd finally get the news. The rumor was: receiving a fat envelope meant that you had failed, and the extra papers in the envelope were instructions for retesting. A skinny envelope was a sure "Pass."

Well, when the envelope finally arrived, it was certainly not skinny. My heart sank, and my mind started racing through all the "what-to-do-now?" scenarios. More classes? Retake the tests? Quit?

Nobody had mentioned how fat was "fat", or how skinny was "skinny". This envelope was somewhere in between the two. Pulling the papers out of the envelope—that just happened to be not too fat and not too skinny, but rather just right - revealed the edge of an official looking document – a Nursing License – with my name on it! Pinch me! Make sure I'm awake, and not dreaming all this!

VIRGINIA STATE BOARD OF NURSING

Be it known that

SUSAN MARIE BREEDEN BROOKS

has met all requirements prescribed by the law or by the Board of Nursing ordinances
for professional nurse registration and is therefore entitled to be known as a

Registered Nurse

According to an Act approved July 1, 1970, as amended
In Witness Whereof the said Board has caused this license No. 55551
to be granted and signed by the President and Secretary of the State Board of Nursing
and attested by its official Seal at Richmond, Virginia
this 11th. day of September 19 74

_____ R. N.
PRESIDENT

_____ R. N.
EXECUTIVE SECRETARY

There it was! A new journey began, but not quite as I had hoped.

My Heart's Desire

I n three years time, God had transformed my nursing "nevers" into my heart's only desire – to work in the NICU – Neonatal Intensive Care Unit. But to my chagrin, I was told that I couldn't start there.

Back in the day – sounds like so long ago, and I guess it was – nursing school graduates were required to work on a medical/surgical unit for at least a year before they could be a staff member in a specialized field of nursing. So, in 1974, as a new graduate, I was hired to work on a GYN medical/surgical floor – doing what I had to, in order to work my way into a specialty area. Not my choice, but nursing was still my calling. I must admit, as hard as it was, I learned a lot from the seasoned nurses there. It was a great place to start, but my heart was set on the NICU.

One afternoon as I was punching the time clock at the end of my day shift, there was an overhead announcement for a Pediatric Resident Inservice on Neonatal Intubation starting at 3pm. Perfect timing for me. I had just signed off from work, and I was free to go! With lightning speed, I made it to the conference room. Taking a deep breath before entering, I slipped into the back of the room hoping to not be noticed. What was I thinking? Dressed in a nursing uniform, I would not be inconspicuous in a room full of doctors. I was approached by a man who inquired as to who

I was and why I was there. Sheepishly I gave him my name, and told him that I thought this inservice would be good information to have for working in the NICU. Next, he asked why I wasn't working in the NICU? To which I replied, "There isn't a position." His response rocked my world. "There is now. Anyone who would come to an inservice like this on their own time, should be where they want to work." That stately gentleman, by the way, just happened to be the Chief Neonatologist for the Unit. The red tape was cut, and the door to the NICU flew open wide for me. Who knew that in one meeting, one encounter would change my life and my career forever? God orchestrates those kinds of events to place people where He calls them to be. He's a God who moves mountains. He certainly moved obstacles that day!

Technological Advances and Constants

Medicine has come a long way since the 1970's – new techniques, advanced and more sophisticated medical equipment, greater knowledge – all to improve the care and outcome for the preterm infants. The Neonatal field exploded with a constant barrage of new procedures dictating the most up to date methods to provide the least invasive, most effective care. The technology was an ever-evolving tool that opened the way for survival of some of our smallest patients.

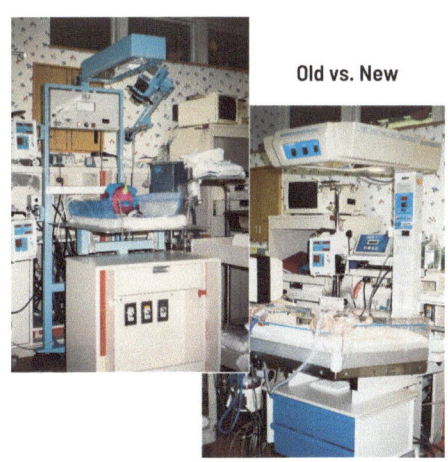

Old vs. New

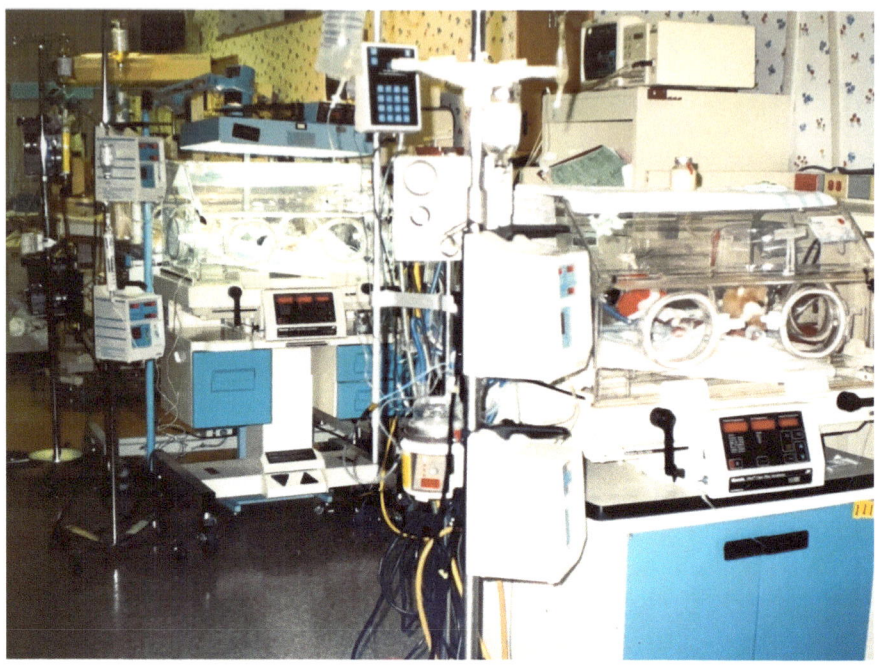

Snapshot of my world

There was always more to learn from our little NICU warriors who signaled us to their bedside with alarms. More technology required more continuing education. Change became the constant. The nurses had to work as a team, staying focused on each individual patient and the task at hand. Embracing change became not only the norm, but an expectation! That doesn't leave any time, or room, for boredom.

Ms Edith Sachs, our most seasoned nurse, taught me a lot of things about "change", and "constants". She exemplified embracing change. Still working when she was in her 80s, she was the mentor for thousands of new nurses and residents. The Nursery was her life, and to anyone who entered the door of the unit, she would greet them with a smile, and say, "Welcome to The Garden Spot of the Hospital." That greeting was a constant!

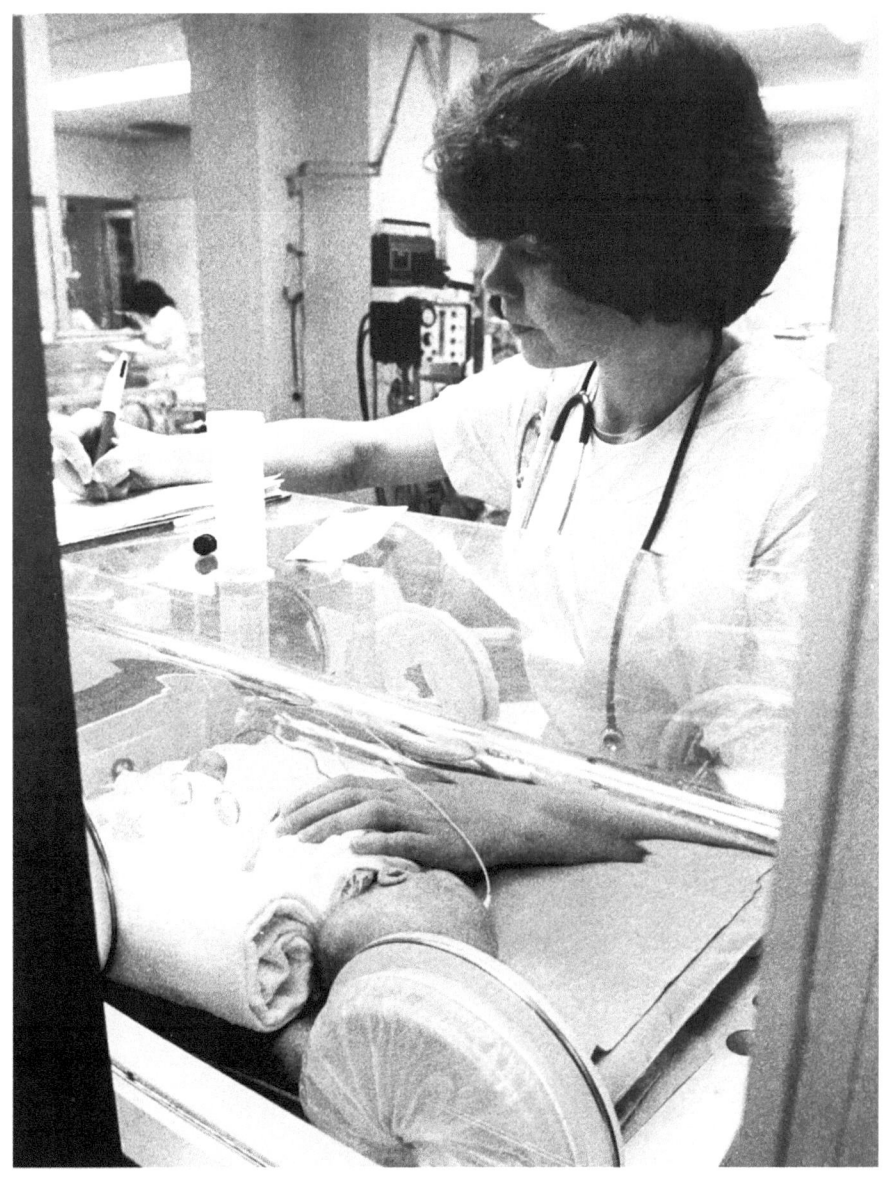

SUSAN STIVER

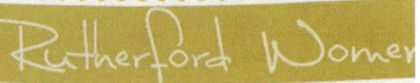

Photos & Interviews By Amy Owens

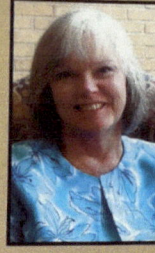

If ever there was a voice for babies, it is **Sue Stiver.** A registered nurse for the past 37 years, Sue spent 22 of those years working with sick babies in the Neonatal Intensive Care Unit. This Rutherford Woman has been at the Cleveland Regional Medical Center for 14 years. She has developed a new protocol to help sick babies heal faster. The protocol is a minimal stimulation process referred to as "Shhh" (for soft lights, hushed tones, help, heal). The study was completed with the help of a fellow worker and support from her husband at home.

Sue knew in her heart that working with babies is what she was meant to do. The new protocol is aimed to help transition sick babies within their local hospital as opposed to transferring them to a major hospital. It is achieved by modifying existing methods of infant care into more calming and effective methods. This transition-versus-transfer theory causes less stress for the baby, and also keeps families together.

While Your
Special Baby
Is In
Our Special Care

A Parents' Guide

Dedicated to Andrew and Cade-Michael
And their Families

Making A Difference

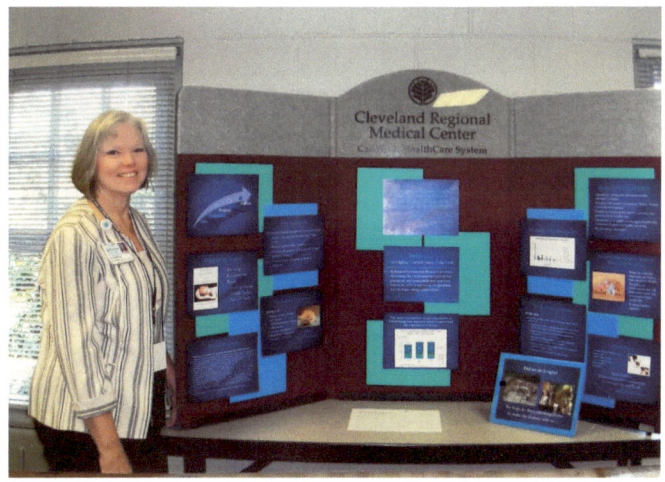

What a pleasure and privilege it was to orchestrate research demonstrating that modifying the environment, and decreasing the noise levels in the Special Care Nursery helped our little patients transition more smoothly to extrauterine life and improved their outcome. Noise equals stress to these newborns who are born prematurely, or are sick at birth. A Minimal Stimulation Policy was developed and implemented. Our babies began to thrive. The transfer rate to tertiary units was reduced by nearly 50%. That, coupled with skin-to-skin contact with the parents, was a win-win for both the babies and the parents. Bonding was promoted, and the parents were involved with their infant's care. Nurses became advocates for this voiceless population. Care providers and parents became a team, and barriers were brought down.

Little did I know the research paper that I had written in Nursing School titled "Let Them Touch: Parental Involvement in the Care of Their High-Risk Infant" would be the foundation for this published accomplishment thirty-seven years later.

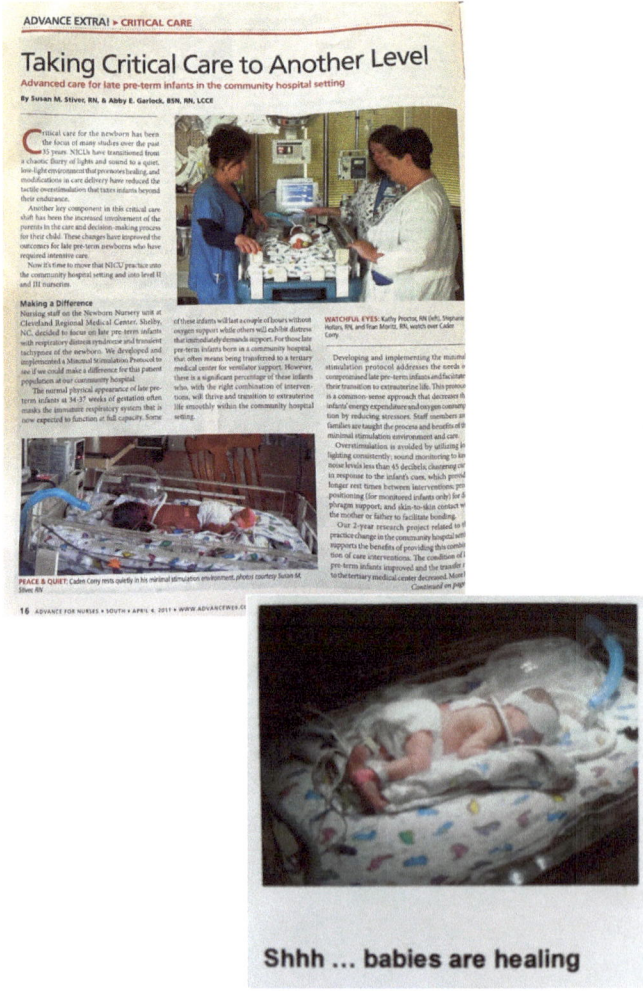

Shhh ... babies are healing

All Roses?

L ife is good, but not always a bed of roses. And even roses have thorns. The best we can do is lean into God, and learn how to navigate through the garden of life.

In this day and time many people can now work from their homes, and have little contact with other company employees. Even some factions of the medical field can do virtual visits and consultations. Not so when it comes to providing the intensive care required for preterm, and sick infants. That level of care demands the cohesiveness of a dedicated team of individuals along with the latest updates in technology. There are struggles, but in this critical care environment, the professionals have to be able to lay down their differences in order to accomplish the task at hand for the good of the patient. Having worked in numerous teaching hospitals in three different states, I can say the challenges were astronomical, but the rewards were far greater! Our little ones received the TLC they needed, and reaped the benefits. It was my privilege to work alongside so many gifted and dedicated professionals who truly did put the patients first!

Throughout my life I have used poetry to express thoughts and queries.
Some poems were written in an effort to reset priorities and focus -
Not just for me, but also for those around me.
In my Nursing Career, it was a way to bring us all
back to center as a team.

Wart Removal

Every place has its warts.
  I can think of one or two.
Let your mind go wander
  To some things that bother you.

Slow down now! Take a break!
  Your list is much too long.
Look again, but closer now –
  Could all this be so wrong?

Change your focus. This time seek
  All things good and right.
Don't forget to count the things
  Far beyond our sight.

Is there food upon your table?
  And a roof above your head?
Does someone feel much better
  From a kind word that you've said?

Did your smile make someone else
  Share that smile throughout the day?
Did you help another walk
  Across a bumpy way?

  Evaluate your findings.
    Answer two questions to be sure –
  "Am I part of the problem?"
    Or "Am I part of the cure?"

  When complaints begin to flow,
    Stop every now and then.
  Take an inner look and ask,
    "Am I the wart again?"

Out of Line

What are you here for?
        The sport? Or the Game?
A pat on the back?
        The money? The fame?
Is it bills to be paid?
        Or a "want" to be bought?
Is it for the challenge
        Of the traffic you've fought?
What are you here for?
        Adult conversation?
A chance to co-mingle
        With the opposite persuasion?
Is it just to catch up
        On your reading or sleep?
Is it really worth it
        for the hours you keep?

                What are you here for?
                        Is there something you missed?
                Is "patient care"
                        Anywhere on your list?
                Were it not for the patient
                        Where would you be?
                The family is counting
                        On you and on me.
                They want some compassion –
                        Is all of yours gone?
                What are you here for?
                        Is it time to move on?

Women Only

Women are so caddy and rude.

    Aren't we glad we're not "one"?

With their arrogant attitudes –

    They scrutinize everyone.

Who do they think they are? –

    Their perfection worn on their sleeve.

Oh, that we could be above reproach,

    Such a perfect life to lead.

It must be lonely at the top

    Looking down on everyone else.

Let's all climb up to perch on high.

    Make room up there on the shelf.

The climb was steep, but we made it.

    Now far as the eye can see

Are a bunch of "perfect" people.

    Could that include you and me?

Where are the "less than perfect"?

    Where could all of them be?

There's no one left beneath the shelf.

    Where are the "scrutinizees"?

Now who can be complained about?

Could there be something else to do?

What about trying some compliments?

What a concept to introduce...

Yes, who do we really think we are,

When negative is all we see?

Have you walked past a mirror today?

Oops, that's not you, it's ME.

Let's all take a look in the mirror
Then compliment each other.

Goodbye to an Outstanding Doctor

Leaving is not an easy thing,
*   Not something one does every day.*
And there's some things we'd like to voice
*   Now that you're on your way.*
We'll think of you when times get rough,
*   And good help's hard to find;*
When we need a reliable sitter –
*   One who doesn't seem to mind.*
We'll think of you in good times
*   When we all shared laughter here;*
And even in some "not-so-good" times
*   When a non-sterile controlled delivery is feared.*
We'll miss the teaching that you've done,
*   The experiences we've shared,*
The many hours you spent with us
*   And all because you cared.*
And yes, we'll miss your yelling,
*   And your favorite little phrase –*
"You Dummy" will not be forgotten
*   Especially on hectic days.*
I could name so many other things
*   That we will miss you for,*
But all those things that I could name
*   Will make us miss you more.*

What Are You Here For?

What is your passion in Nursing?

      Are you here for a cure, or the cause?

Are you here for the recognition,

      Or the sound of the roaring applause?

Are you here to treat whatever ails you?

      Is the job just a means to an end?

What are you really here for?

      Examine your motives, my friend.

We're looked to for healing and comfort

      By those who are helpless and hurt.

It's all about them, and not about us –

      The patient has to come first!

Expensive Cuts

Every now and then do you ever wonder

      What goes on in the land down under?

No, not Australia, or under the sea...

      It's the bowel of the hospital – SPD.

Who got our shipment of unpowdered gloves,

      Our white paper towels, and our orders of...

Softnets to care for our infants' skin,

      Hefty trash bags for all our bins?

Last but not least, can you figure out why

      We only have <u>half</u> of what should be two-ply?

But that's not the last of our very least,

      The source of the problem, or the heart of the beast!

To be "cost effective" is frugal and wise,

      But they're cutting the staff like they're cutting supplies!

Let's look at the math – complete the equation:

      Two minus one plus management evasion...

Equals a shortage, with a load hard to bear,

      Paperwork a plenty, and no time to care.

If you or your family just happen to be

    The patient who's waiting, be patient with me.

Know that my heart has a burden to care,

    And as soon as I can, I'll rush to be there.

Don't blink or you'll miss me, as I come running through.

    Please know in my heart – I DO care about you.

<u>Life Goes On</u> —

Where do friends take you
*   When the bottom falls out?*
To the Rock Bottom Restaurant –
*   A brewery, no doubt.*

Not to drink beer
*   Or drown in your sorrow –*
But to tell funny stories
*   And plan for tomorrow.*

A Belly Dance Class
*   At the crack of dawn?*
We talked about life
*   Till the evening was gone.*

No time to bemoan
*   The hurt and the pain –*
With inside-out umbrellas
*   We laughed through the rain.*

Back to the Hotel
*   For a good night of rest.*
Friendships like these
*   Are truly the best!*

Proverbs 17:22 A joyful heart is good medicine.

Tara, Tonya, Deborah, and Frieda
Thank you for being there for me in a strange city, a long way from
home. I thank God for the gift of our friendships.
Milwaukee, WI/October 1, 2010

Challenge By Choice

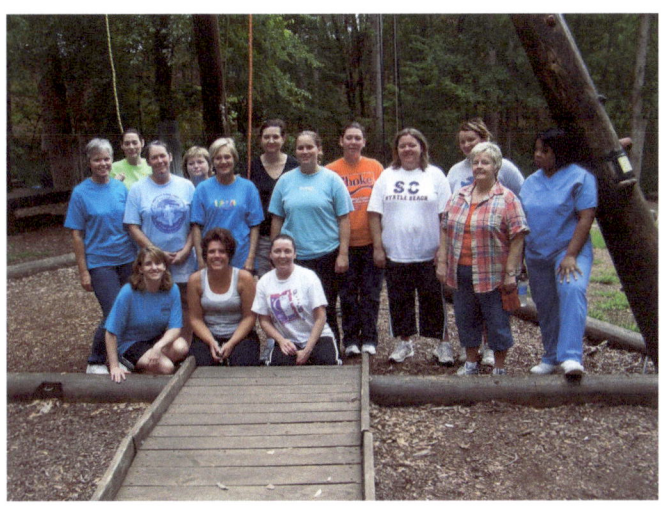

"Challenge by choice" –
*   And challenged we were.*
Who would go first?
*   Was it me? Was it her?*
Strapped in a harness,
*   Strung by a rope,*
Climbing to heights –
*   The "belay on" my hope.*
"Climb on" – the command,
*   And climb on we did –*
Each to her own goal.
*   We climbed – no one hid.*
Some pulled, and some pushed,
*   Some took up the slack.*
Once on the way up –
*   There was no turning back.*
We cheered, and we clapped,
*   We watched, and we gazed.*

🐦

As the tower was topped –
    We stood there amazed.
Then "climb on" we did,
    First one, then another –
We conquered the tower
    By helping each other.
Is life any different
    Than a tower so tall?
Tie the knots, check your harness –
    Let's go climb some walls!

Dedicated to the **Climb Team** of Nurses from the Women's and Children's Services Department at CRMC

Mandy —

When the sun comes up
And your day begins –
Remember the nights
And remember your friends.

Remember the popcorn
And microwave ablaze.
Remember the rescue.
You'll miss us on days.

Remember the stories
That made us all friends.
Know that we'll be here
When your day shift ends.

P.S. Who will sing for you?

How Did We Do It?

Written for all the nurses I worked with over the years

Who could know the depths
    of love it would take
To work side by side
    For the patient's sake?

Yet through all the turmoil,
    The haves and have-nots,
We locked arms together
    Through all the hard spots.

I covered your back,
    And you covered mine.
Triumphant we made it,
    Time after time.

Sometimes with laughter,
    Sometimes through tears,
We overcame obstacles
    And conquered our fears.

How gallant and brave

    We all seemed to be.

We fought hard for life,

    And each little one's needs.

The needs overrode

    The differences we had.

We worked as if one

    Through the good and the bad.

I look back with pride

    For all we came through.

Our passion was life,

    And I'm grateful for you.

Little Voices

When words can't be spoken, hearts have a way of breaking through the
silence to connect with each other. Forty years spent in the Neonatal
(Newborn) world taught me volumes about love,
heart-to-heart communication, and the life-giving power of touch.
Each life is a precious gift and priceless treasure.

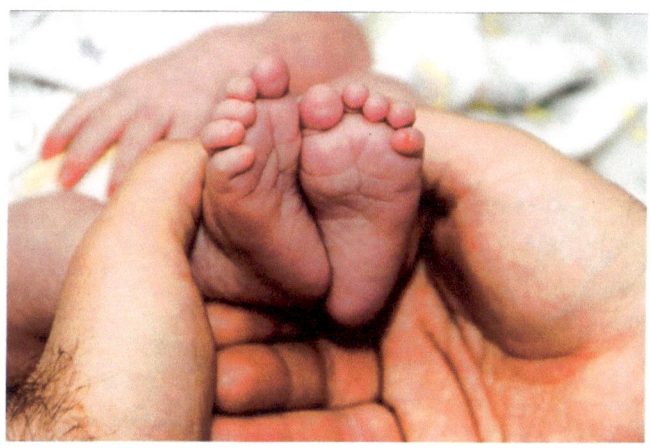

Dedicated to the Little Ones
Who fought for their lives as NICU Warriors,
and to their families
who endured the pain and struggles
along side them.

On the Outside Looking In

Telling the NICU story would be incomplete without including what it looks like from the parents' perspective.

I can testify to the scary part – going through denial, feeling helpless and detached. Even having been a NICU nurse, for nine years at that time, didn't prepare me for seeing my baby lying on the warmer, hooked up to monitors and IVs. That had to be someone else's baby, not mine. But she was mine, and that day changed me as a NICU nurse. My work had always focused exclusively and intensively on the babies. Now I understood the needs of the parents. I felt what they felt and could better relate to their struggle. It wasn't just the baby fighting for its life – it was a family fighting a battle for life.

What's a Few More Days?

What's a few more days to mother,
  When months have come and gone?
What's one more day to walk away,
  And go home all alone?
What's one more hour in the house,
  To rock with empty arms?
What's one more minute without her child?
  What could be the harm?

It's a few more days to mother
  In a world that's dark and drear.
It's one more day to walk away
  Leaving part of herself here.
It's one more hour to sit and think
  Of how things might have been.
It's one more minute without her child –
  An eternity without end!

I have invited other parents to share their stories.

Michael & Ashlee's Story

WRITTEN BY ASHLEE REED

H ello! Our names are Michael and Ashlee Reed. Our story is a wild adventure that has been touched by God's hand with every unexpected twist and turn. We were married in March of 2020, right as the COVID-19 lockdown was starting. Due to the restrictions on how large gatherings could be, we had to change our wedding timeline from having 120 guests in April 2020 to 10 guests in March of that year. We ended up getting married, going on our honeymoon and moving all in the same weekend.

We are both family-oriented people so we knew we wanted to start trying to have a family shortly after we got married. After suffering a miscarriage, we decided to apply to become foster-to-adopt parents. Only 10 days after putting in our application, we found out we were pregnant again! So, for 9 months, we had a parallel journey of pregnancy and becoming foster parents. Early in our pregnancy, we found out we were having a little boy, so we requested to foster a little girl, so we could have one of each gender.

Our world got turned upside down when we learned at the 20-week anatomy ultrasound appointment that our son Judah had an Omphalocele, which is like a sac with some of the organs from his abdominal cavity lying above his stomach instead of inside his tummy where it should be.

We were told he would have to have surgery during the first few weeks of his life, but that hopefully he would go on to lead a normal life. We were initially devastated and horrified at the idea of our tiny newborn having to go under the knife. After meeting with many specialists and having a slew of appointments it was decided that it would be safest for Judah to enter the world via C-Section on May 4, 2022.

Judah was a beautiful little boy with a head full of curly black hair. Before he was placed on heavy sedatives, he tried to lift his head to see myself and Michael when we came to greet him in the NICU. Immediately upon arrival, the Doctors were concerned about Judah's ability to breathe on his own because he had a severe case of Pulmonary Hypoplasia. His lungs were too small and underdeveloped for him to be able to sustain his own blood pressure. He was transferred to a Children's Hospital when he was about 24 hours old. Upon arrival, they told us that he was not a good candidate for ECMO (a heart-lung bypass machine that would breathe for him) because it could cause him to have a brain bleed. They said there was nothing they could do for him. In our desperation, we called Michael's spiritual father and asked him to pray for Judah. That same hour that he prayed, Judah's vital signs started to improve. The Doctors were amazed that he was still alive days after the grim prognosis. Since he responded so well, Michael began doing live videos on social media asking for people to pray for Judah. Judah lived long enough to be baptized on his 8th day of life and to be prayed for by over 2k people all over the world. Although he passed away on May 13, 2022, we had multiple reports that his short time on earth had reignited people's faith and trust in God.

After he passed, we told our case manager that we were open to adopting any child, whether they were medically fragile or not. We felt like we were about to go all in for Judah, so why not become great parents for another child who is medically fragile? Sensing our need to parent a young child, our case manager placed us with a beautiful 2 yr old little girl who was ready to be adopted. Our daughter was truly a godsend because I believe Michael and I needed a little one to hold in our arms and rock to sleep at night.

As we were going through our grieving process, we reflected on how difficult the process had been to navigate the NICU, where to stay in an unfamiliar city while our child was in the hospital, how to look up resources for a medically fragile child, etc. We decided we wanted to offer a place for medically fragile children to live who didn't have parents who could advocate, or care, for them. There are many children who need around the clock medical care, but there are few resources for them in our area. Michael and I created a non-profit organization called Warrior Restoration. Our goal is to provide housing to medically fragile children who need 24-hour medical attention. Michael is currently in nursing school and hopes to get his doctorate, so that he can help medically fragile children just like Judah to thrive no matter their diagnosis. We are hopeful that it will be a place where prayer happens constantly and miracles happen regularly in the lives of some of God's most precious treasures.

We would be delighted for anyone to reach out. If you would like more information about Warrior Restoration, please call Michael or Ashlee Reed at 540-314-5811 or email us at Ashlee.murphy32@gmail.com.

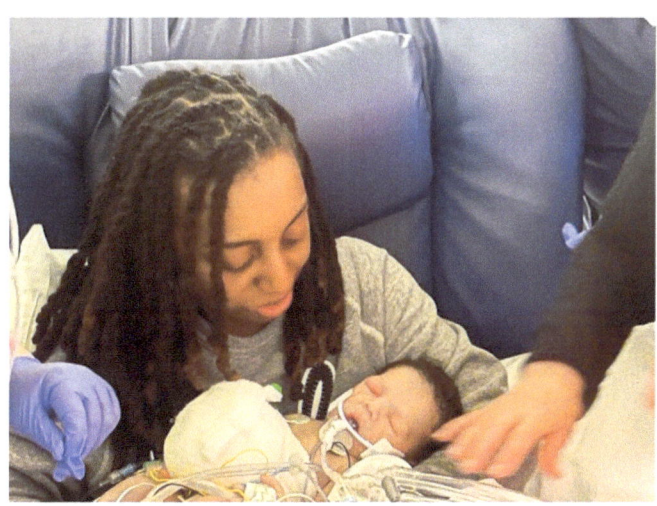

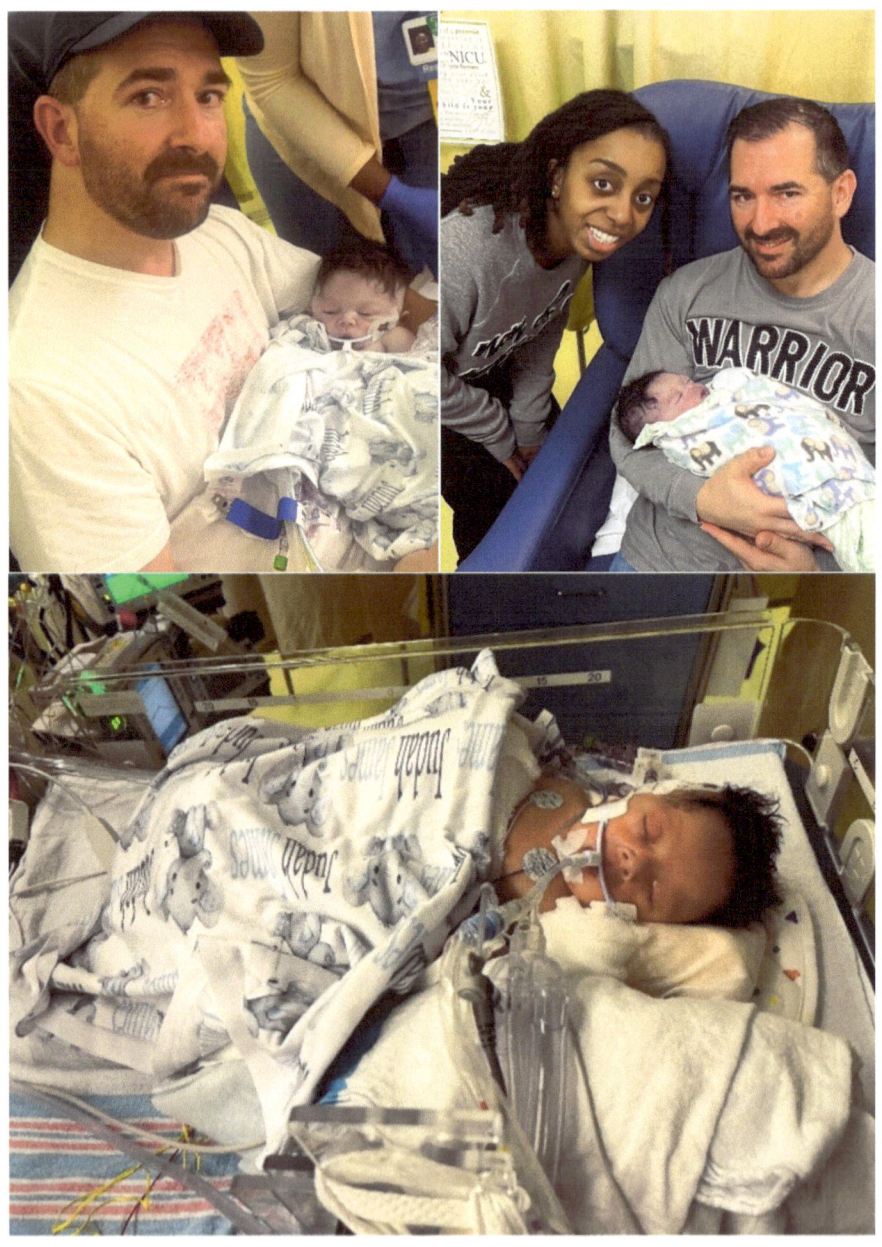

Little NICU Warrior

Little NICU Warrior,
*   Brave and fearless one,*
I wish I were as brave as you
*   When all is said and done.*

You came into a world
*   So unlike your own –*
A place so big and frightful,
*   But you were not alone.*

People all around you
*   Did their best to help you through,*
But there was Someone greater
*   Taking care of you.*

He held your hand and whispered,
*   "You are my special child.*
I'll fight this battle for you."
*   And then in love, He smiled.*

The battle raged around you,
*   And in His tender care,*
He wrapped you in your parents' arms –
*   No safer place than there.*

Rest there, Little Warrior,
*   Close to your parents' heart.*
They are your armor bearers –
*   That's their special part.*

With special dedication to Judah James Reed,

and his parents Michael and Ashlee.

Nothing Short of a Miracle - Holden's Story

WRITTEN BY HIS MOTHER, CHRISTINA LAFON

Our son is living a life today that would not have been possible apart from a miracle. There had been no complications during my pregnancy or the repeat C-Section delivery, and Holden arrived on time. Aside from a mild heart murmur, of no concern to the doctors, Holden had been a perfectly healthy baby, nursing well and sleeping as expected. His one-week check-up went well.

Everything changed on his eighth day of life. My sister-in-law had picked me and the kids up for dinner at her house. Ashlyn, my daughter was almost three, and Holden just a week old. Dinner was great with family and friends all around. After our visit, my sister-in-law drove us home, and offered to help me get the kids ready for bed. She was a pro with four children of her own. Managing two little ones was still new to me. Needless to say, I accepted her offer. That was when one of my worst nightmares and biggest miracles began to unfold.

As I was getting Holden ready for bed, he started gagging, going limp, lifeless, and turning blue in my arms. I handed him to my sister-in-law, and told her what had happened. He did it again. She immediately contacted our pastor's wife who was a baby nurse at Mary Black Hospital, she only lived five minutes away. We knew she'd be able to examine him and give us some insight. As we waited, I called 911 in case he needed extra support.

Once the ambulance arrived, they wasted no time giving Holden oxygen support, and transporting him to the nearby hospital. The next thing I remember is God placing a kind and loving nurse in our path, who saw the stress we were under. She tightly hugged us, and asked to pray with us. That is how I met Sue for the first time. When life feels chaotic, God sends reminders to be still and ask for His help. As surprised as I was about my healthy boy having these strange episodes, I am confident God was not caught off guard. He already knew, had everything in place, and was at work all around us.

Holden was admitted to a room on the Pediatric floor, placed on oxygen and a monitor. I was able to take a nap there until around 2am. Then it happened again – Holden had another episode. The nurses did what they could for him, but there was still a problem. They reached out to the Pediatric Doctor on call. She diligently stood at the bedside table in our dimly lit room flipping through the biggest resource book I'd ever laid eyes on. The Doctor determined this was one of two heart defects, both of which are correctable with surgery. She was coming up with a plan to save his life. Again, God had put the right person, in the right place, at the right time to guide and help us when we needed it most. In one night, He'd orchestrated my sister-in-law to be with me, the pastor's wife to be at home to help, the ambulance workers to have wisdom, a nurse to cover us in prayer, and now the Doctor on call to help transition us to the next steps.

It wasn't long before Holden had another more severe episode. His oxygen level dropped down to the 30s, and he began gagging again. This time I had to step out of the room as the hospital alarm sounded, and every available Doctor ran into his room. He had coded. Once they were able to get a handle on his oxygen levels, they knew they had to get him to a larger hospital equipped to handle his condition as soon as possible. They needed him stable enough to move, but had to get him moved regardless. The helicopter was called, but was not available, so we got in an ambulance around daybreak and headed to a larger hospital about an hour away. The ambulance driver was calm and kind. He allowed us to be encouraged by Christian radio in the background as we traveled. My sister-in-law rode with me in the front seat, and we were able to keep an eye on Holden with the medical workers in the back.

The ER team was waiting for us outside the Emergency Room entrance when we arrived. They rushed Holden in and ran some tests. The heart Doctors were ready to conference with us within 15-20 minutes. One Surgeon drew a picture of Holden's heart showing us where there were two narrowings in his aorta that would need to be rebuilt in order for him to survive. One narrowing was 1mm and the other was 3mm. They were supposed to be 9mm each. I know God did not make any mistakes in making him. I also knew and believed the same God who had made that tiny heart was capable to supernaturally give him a new one, or could heal him through surgery. Holden was too small to believe, so it was my job to believe for him to receive the miracle he needed. In the Bible, the book of James reminded me that if we don't believe, we should not expect to receive anything from the Lord. I'm sure I did not believe perfectly, but when I found myself doubting, I went back to the Word and chose to put my trust back in God's good plan for Holden's life. Isn't that all God wants from us. Not to live perfectly, but stay in relationship with Him, returning to His loving arms each day as we stray? At that time Jeremiah 29:11 in my mind was for babies (now I know it is for everyone). He had a plan to prosper Holden and had a hopeful future for him.

The Doctors said Holden was very sick with congestive heart failure. He would need surgery. But first he would require a medication to close his PDA. For a few days we prayed that the medication would close the ductus, and that he would be strong enough to undergo open heart surgery.

Those days were intense. I remember watching through the glass in the PICU as they shocked his little body back to life countless times. The elders of the church came in one afternoon to anoint him with oil and pray for his healing. There were countless others from our family, church and community lifting us up in this tragic time, and God heard their prayers of faith.

On the morning of March 20th, the Doctors decided he had a chance to make it through surgery, so they operated. For 10 hours I stayed in the waiting room. I remember a few conversations with the receptionist about what was going on, and at the end of the day telling her he had come through. Hearing the good news, I remember her saying to me, "God is good." I walked out of the waiting room thinking about how true that was. Yes, God IS good, BUT He is still good whether Holden came through surgery or not. Our circumstances do not change an unchanging God who is the same yesterday, today and forever. He is good and I guess you could say that was one of many, many times I visibly saw His goodness running after me.

I will never understand how the Doctors were able to operate on that teeny, tiny heart. I cannot imagine the protection God had over him during that time. To this day, Holden is convinced he sat with God in heaven, and I believe he probably did.

After surgery, they warned us that he would not be out of the woods for several days, so we continued to pray. Most of the time, I didn't know what to pray, but the prayers of others carried us through. We know that the Great Physician saved Holden's life through the doctors. We asked for His healing touch and wisdom for them. God gave both generously.

In recovery for the next 5 weeks, with a 50/50 chance of survival, Holden spent each day with a one-on-one nurse at his bedside. I was only allowed to visit him every two hours for 15 minutes at a time. For six weeks I spent 24 hours at the hospital, and the next 24 hours at home with my 3-year-old daughter, rotating my days and nights. When at the hospital, I slept in the waiting rooms. Day and night I set my alarm to visit him every two hours to get all of the possible visits in before driving the hour and a half back home.

When I was with Holden, I touched him and kissed him even though other visitors were told it was not allowed. I talked to him about what we would do when he came home, and prayed for his recovery. At times I knew it would still be a while, and I told him it would be best to wait and come home when it was warmer. I wanted us to think and believe for better days ahead. It was a tough road, to say the least. In order to get to his heart, the Doctors had to break his sternum. Post surgery, we prayed diligently for 11 days for the swelling to go down so they could remove the clear tape covering his heart and close him back up. He looked like a little sumo wrestler with his ears and tongue swollen with all of the excess fluid.

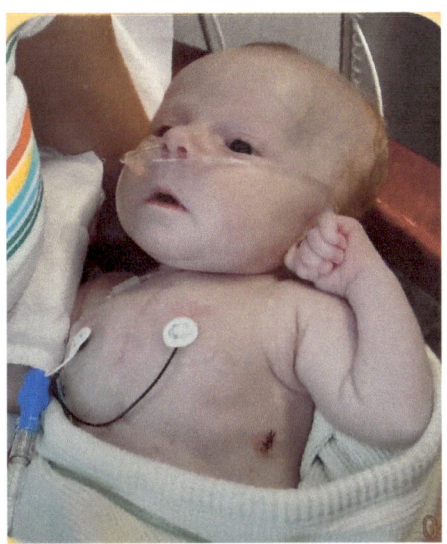

I know God was with him and protected him each and every moment. Finally, the time came to move into a regular room. Holden learned to nurse again after having a feeding tube for 5 weeks. A week later, he was discharged on 22 doses of medication, including IV antibiotics that I administered through the night. It was complicated to keep up with, yet imperative that we didn't miss a dose.

Early on we had been told, "He's the least likely to survive based of his gender and race; he won't like being touched or held; he will be on medications for life; he won't be able to play sports; and he will have dark colored baby and adult teeth."

As Holden grew, I often looked back at the poems scribed during those difficult days, trusting the line that tells me, one day he'll proclaim his testimony as a man. Those poems are hanging on his bedroom wall, and here we are 17 years later. Holden has not required any additional surgeries since he was about 3 months old. He did get a chance at life. He is very loving, and has always enjoyed physical touch. His teeth have been perfect in every way, and he's not been on any medications since he was an infant. He has been able to play the sports he wanted with no restrictions. We are so thankful that Jesus made a way, and let Ashlyn keep her little brother. God had, and still has, a good plan for his life, and He will finish what He started in each of us as He promised. God has been our Healer since then, and still is in so many ways. We've seen, and will remember, the miracles He has done, and we trust Him for the next.

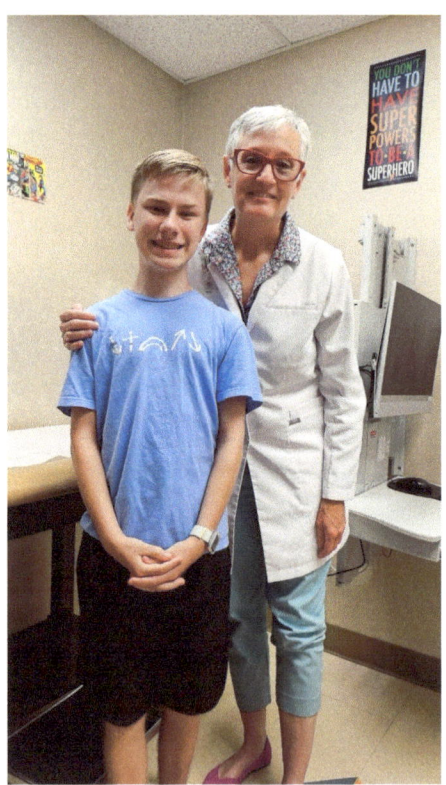

God always provides, always helps, and is always with us. I am thankful in more ways than one that He is close to the brokenhearted. It's also been reassuring to me that God is never caught off guard. Because of this one incident, I've never had to wonder or worry about the people I love. I remember that night Holden needed Him the most. He came through in every way throughout this tragedy that turned into a miracle, and He always will because He is a God that never changes.

Holden's Letter

Dear Mom and Dad,

Some say we're all born with a hole in our heart
        That only God can fill.
Mine is of a different kind,
        But I know He loves me still.

As my Maker and my Father
        He knows my every part.
It is no surprise to Him
        That I have a special heart.

By His design He formed me –
        A masterpiece to be sure.
He has plans for even me –
        A future that's secure.

I'm not exactly sure what that means,
        But I know to trust His plan,
Because He whispers deep within my heart,
        And holds me in His hand.

That hole that is within me –
        God has filled it to the brim
With love for you my parents
        And abiding love for Him.

So as you sit beside me
        And gaze into my face,
Read the love God has for us
        That transcends all time and space.

Holden's Second Letter

Mom, I have a testimony
       Even as little as I am.
Every day of life is a miracle –
       One day I'll proclaim it as a man.

God's teaching me to wait on Him –
       He holds me in His hand.
He whispers softly in my ears –
       And tells me all His plans.

He's given me eyes to see your face,
       And ears to hear your voice.
He's given me hands to feel your touch –
       He makes my heart rejoice.

I've seen your tears and heard your cry,
       I know you've seen mine too.
Our Father God has seen us both
       And has heard both me and you.

So as you sit beside me
       Know that He's wrapped you in His arms.
He cradles us like Fathers do
       To keep us safe from harm.

Now rest with me in Daddy's care.
       Take comfort in that place.
Know that I love you very much –
       Read my heart and then my face.

I love you, Mommy.

Our Baby Boy

WRITTEN BY HIS MOTHER, KIM MARKS

September 25, 1997 was a day of excitement for our family. Our third son was to be born that day. We had prepared for our baby's birth for nine long months. Everything had gone according to plan until I was diagnosed with Gestational Diabetes. I was so scared and had no idea what to expect along the way. I followed my diet and tried to do everything right, but my glucose readings were still out of control. My doctors felt it best for me to be put on insulin. I took four to five shots a day depending on my glucose reading. The insulin made me feel terrible, but I tried hard not to let it show.

Because of the diabetes I had to go to the doctor for sonograms and stress tests twice weekly near the end of my pregnancy. Many times, between the visits, I would have to call the doctor, and let them know I hadn't felt the baby move very much, or not at all. The remedy prescribed was to drink a Diet Sundrop and lay on my left side. If I didn't feel him move within 30 minutes I was to go to the hospital. He moved every time. What a relief. Thank you, God, for taking care of us.

Then our big day came. Due to the Gestational Diabetes, I would need to have my labor induced. Wow, that was such a change after having two other pregnancies with no issues. I just wanted my baby to be healthy. We arrived at the hospital at 6:00am on the morning of Thursday, September 25, 1997. Scared to death, but we were so ready to know that everything was okay. My labor was induced and progressed nicely, and at 11:11am, our sweet baby boy, Andrew Hunter Marks was born. The sound of that cry was music to our ears. He was healthy, strong and absolutely precious. Ten fingers, ten toes, and our prayers had been answered. Later that day, our sweet baby would meet his two brothers, who were ready to play and show him everything they knew about how to get into mischief.

We settled into our room getting ready for the nursery nurse to bring the baby to our room. Instead, the nurse knocked on our door, and had some very disturbing news to deliver. Andrew had been given some glucose water in the nursery to help his blood sugar level, and he had some difficulties. He had stopped breathing and turned blue. Of course, they did everything possible to get him through the crisis, and he now was under an Oxy hood, on a heart monitor, and had an IV. There was no medical explanation for why this happened at this point, everything had been perfectly normal since delivery. The doctors ordered numerous tests, and consulted with doctors at another hospital. Still no explanation, every test was normal. There was talk of transferring Andrew to a NICU unit at another hospital if needed, but there was no diagnosis, no abnormality in the tests. The nurses were so good to us. They allowed us to go into the nursery frequently just to touch his hand, and let him know we were there and that we loved him. The nurses tried several times to lower the oxygen concentration, and remove the oxy hood, but each time, our little bundle of joy couldn't handle it, and his saturation numbers would start to drop. Still no explanation.

I felt so helpless. My husband and I couldn't fix this. What was going to happen? We were devastated, but so blessed by all the compassion and care that was being shown, not only to our precious baby, but also to us. We didn't have to ask for updates or changes in his condition, nurses were in and out of our room continuously keeping us informed. We had so many people taking care of us, yet nothing was changing – WHY? This wasn't supposed to happen.

During this journey, we met Sue Stiver. She, and several other nurses, took so much time, with our little boy. They worked extra shifts and hours so that he would have consistent care – not because they had to, but because they cared about him and us.

The first day of Andrew's life was not what we hoped for, but we knew in our hearts, day two would be better. However, it was not. Nothing worked – oxygen saturations still dropping when his oxygen concentrations were decreased – but all the tests were normal. The nurses were so good to us. We were allowed to go in the Nursery and hold him for a few minutes and feed him his bottles. Day three and four were the same. On the evening of Day four, we were told that all the tests would be repeated, and a determination would be made about transferring us to another facility. We were so scared. What were we facing? We wanted answers – the unknown was unbearable. It was like a very bad dream.

On the morning of Day five, something very unexpected occurred. The tests were repeated, and all were normal. Doctors were making calls to consult with other physicians on next steps. During this time, Andrew became a little rambunctious. It seemed he had squirmed enough to pull his IV out, and his oxygen saturations had increased. He was going to continue to be monitored, but he could actually be brought to our room. He had made a huge change. Still no real explanations of why this happened, but everything was okay.

We were excited that we might get discharged to go home, but we were also a little apprehensive. What if something happened again? During our journey, we met so many wonderful, caring and compassionate nurses and doctors. One of the nurse's mothers even crocheted a blanket for our precious boy. Finally, our time had come – Day six and Andrew was fine. No more issues, oxygen levels and bloodwork were all normal. We were going home.

There were several visits to the doctor's office, just for weight checks and some bloodwork, but everything was great. Our pediatrician shared that Andrew might have some difficulties as he learned to do all the normal things babies do, like rolling over, crawling, walking, talking, but Andrew learned everything right on time, and had no issues. As he grew, he did have some difficulties with asthma type illnesses, but he outgrew those, and has no issues now.

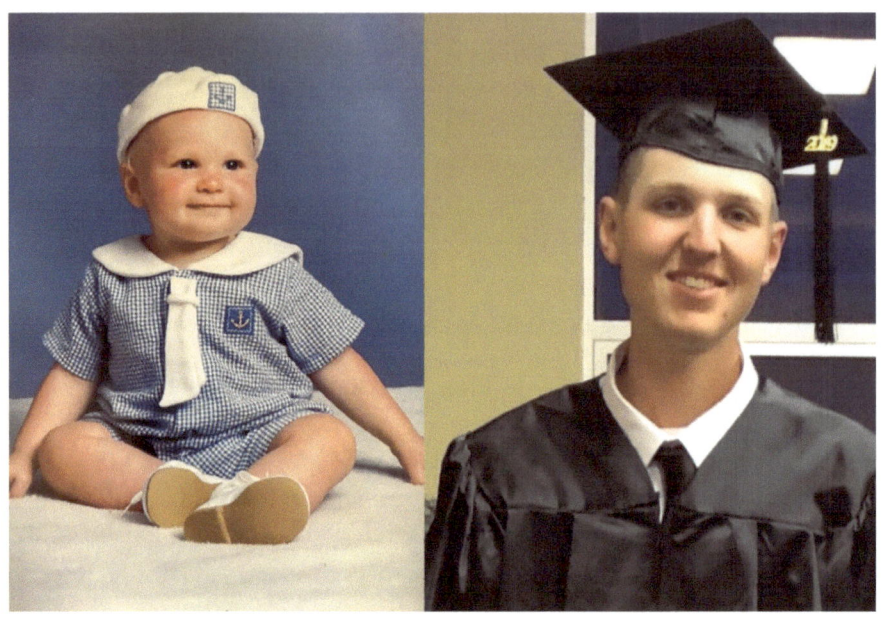

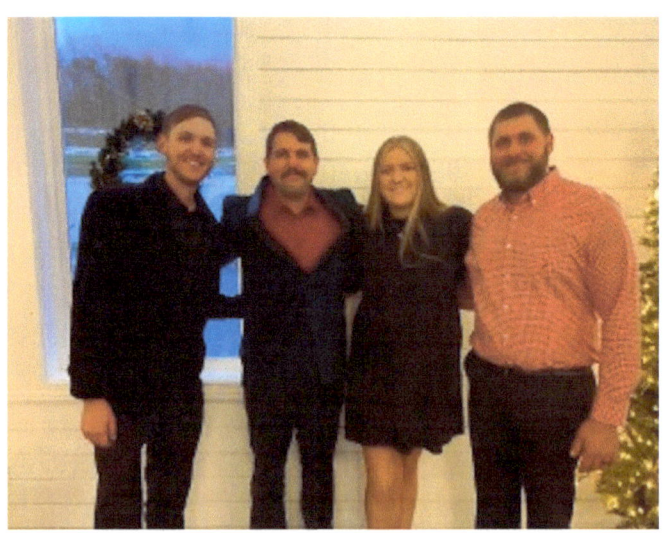

Andrew with his siblings Lucas, Maggie, and Zachery

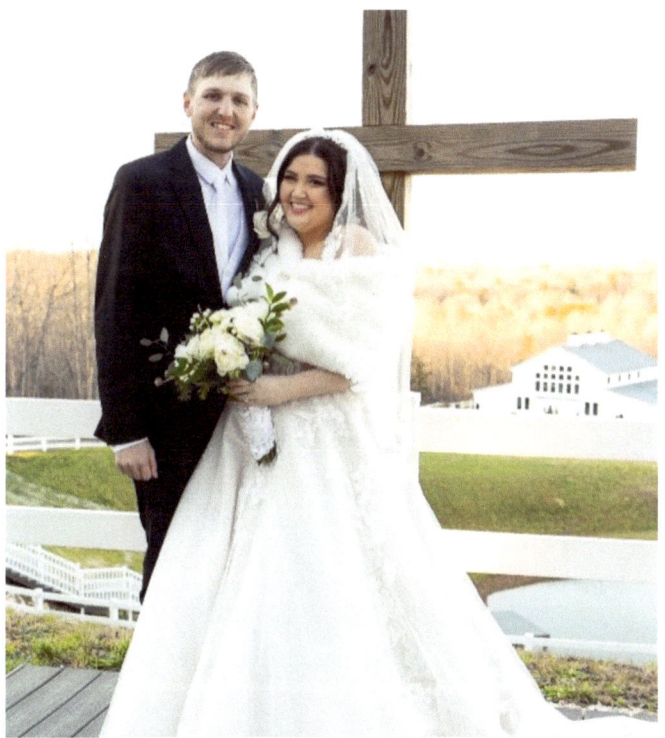

Andrew is now 27 years old, and recently married the love of his life.

A father and mother's dream come true.

Ask the Whys

Why do we parents share our stories? Several reasons. Sometimes, just telling, or writing our story helps us to gather our thoughts and "whys", then from that emerges a broader perspective and greater understanding of the experience. Other times, sharing the story reaches out and touches someone else in need of comfort for what they have been through, or are going through. It can validate that person, and as such, give them permission to voice their story and ask their "whys". Often times, it helps us find answers - even years after the event. With that comes great peace.

Most importantly sharing our stories brings and delivers healing to us and those around us. For anyone who has been down those long hospital halls, know that you were never alone. May God bless you with healing and wholeness. Share your story. Your words are hope and healing for others.

Now may the God of hope fill you with all
joy and peace in believing,
so that you will abound in hope
by the power of the Holy Spirit.
Romans 15:13

Grace to you and peace from God our Father
and the Lord Jesus Christ.
Blessed be the God and Father of our Lord Jesus Christ,
the Father of mercies and God of all comfort,
who comforts us in all our affliction
so that we will be able to comfort those
who are in any affliction
with the comfort with which we ourselves
are comforted by God.
2 Corinthians 1:2-4

A Voice for the Voiceless Newborn

Stand up and be counted!

But suppose I cannot stand?

Wave to get their attention!

But suppose I can't raise my hand?

Articulate what you want!

But suppose I cannot speak?

Cry out with your loudest voice!

But suppose my cry is weak?

Look for those who will help you!

But suppose my eyes can't see?
I've just come from total darkness –
The light's too bright for me.

My world was small and cozy.
The sounds were muffled tones.
Cradled inside my mother's womb –
I never felt alone.

Now my world is upside down –
It's LOUD and BRIGHT! I'm cold!
I'm lost in a world of giants,
And I'm only hours old.

Where's my Mommy? Help me find her.
I'm as frightened as can be.
Is there anybody out here
Who will speak, and cry out for me?

- Voiceless Newborn

"Speak up for those who cannot speak for themselves."

Proverbs 31:8 NIV

The Whispers and Cries of the Newborn

Hear the whispers and cries of the newborns
who dictated words of love in letters to their parents
as scribed by me their care provider.

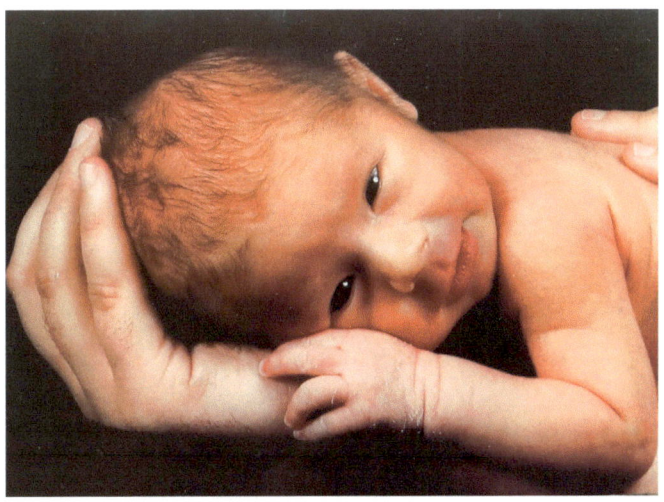

Unspoken Words from Me to You

I can't speak, but I know you're there.
      Standing beside me, I know you care.
That troubled look upon your face
      Says more to me than time and space.
I can see, you know, it hurts me, too,
      To see that I have troubled you.
I cry because I have no voice.
      All this sorrow was not my choice.
Please talk to me, your voice is dear.
      Thank you for your time spent here.
I only wish that you could know
      How much I love and need you so.

Even From a Distance

Dear Mom and Dad,

Thank you for staying near me
    Did you know I can hear your heart?
I hear it when you hold me,
    And even when we're apart.

It's really quite amazing –
    No matter far or near,
God has knit our hearts as one -
    So to me you're always here.

Without a word I know your thoughts.
    I think you know mine, too.
With every breath of every day
    We whisper "I love you".

That's a special gift between us
    That didn't happen just by chance.
God knit our hearts to beat as one –
    Even when it's from a distance.

I love you.

Carli's Letter

Every day is different –
New faces and new routines.
But in these constant changes
There are some constant things.

The sun will rise and night will fall,
But most importantly...
You will come with daylight,
And rock me lovingly.

Secure in knowing you will come,
I will wait for you...
Because there is another constant
And that's my love for you.

Denzel's Letter

A Mother's a special person –
    No one can take her place.
No one can read me a story,
    Or wear that sweet smile on her face.

No one's as gentle and loving.
    No one can sing so sweet.
No one can bathe me like she does,
    Or clothe me with socks on me feet.

Nurses are nice and they're helpful.
    Their TLC will do in a pinch.
I love them, but not like my Mommy -
    She wins hands down. It's a cinch!

No choice to be made. No contest.
    Mother, you're one of a kind.
In all the world, I'm the luckiest boy,
    Because dear Mommy, you're mine!

Emory's Letter

Dear Mom and Dad,

I'm sorry if I scared you
    By coming out too soon.
August 2nd was too far off –
    So I chose the 5th of June.

I couldn't wait to see your face
    And be held in your arms,
So in my haste I came early....
    I didn't mean to cause alarm.

I'll do my best to grow quickly,
    And make you proud of me.
I hope and pray you're better than I
    At waiting patiently.

Marissa's Letter

Dear Mom and Dad

Remember the night you sat with me
    And rocked me oh so lovingly?
    - I do.

Remember holding me so close to your heart
    And how I really liked that part?
    - I do.

Remember how gently you kissed my head
    When I lay helpless in my bed?
    - I do.

Remember your tear that touched my face
    When we were both lost in time and space?
    - I do.

Remember having to be apart
    For any length of time?
    - I don't.
I only know that through it all
    Your hearts were tied to mine.

Leigh's Letter

Dear Mom and Dad, If I could speak
    There's so much I would say.
First, I'd say "I love you!
    Thanks for coming every day!"
Then I'd thank the Lord above
    For giving me to you.
You're very special parents,
    And I know you love me, too.
I see your smiles and hear your voice.
    I know your gentle touch.
I know by everything you do
    That you love me very much.
I feel your sense of worry.
    I know how much you care.
What a comfort it is to me
    Just knowing that you're there.
Now and then I see that tear
    You so bravely try to hide.
Thank you for being strong for me,
    And being by my side.
But I understand if you should cry,
    I know they're tears of love.
They reach the very Heavens
    And touch the heart of God.
If I could speak, there'd be no words
    To express my love for you.
So, from heart to heart, we'll communicate
    As children and parents do.

The Circle

There is a Family Circle
    Complete within itself
That's seen in generations
    Of pictures on a shelf.

It's a sacred kind of circle
    The outside dare not breach,
With walls so high and fortified –
    The entrance out of reach.

Then something special happens
    And the circle must expand –
It's the very gift of life itself
    And another pair of hands.

But he came a little early
    Jon Gavin couldn't wait!
He just had to see his Mom and Dad –
    So, he moved up the date!

January twenty-fourth
    Sure looked good to him,
So, he made his entrance,
    And the circle grew again.

The circle engulfed the nurses
    As they shared the tears and joy.
The gift is now a blessing!
    And the celebration – It's a Boy!

William and Walter's Letter

Dear Mom and Dad

Thank you for holding us
    close to your heart.
We knew that you loved us
    right from the start.

Thank you for every
    tear you shed,
And for all the kisses
    on our heads.

Thank you for love
    whispered in our ears.
Our skin was sprinkled
    with your tears.

Please know that
    we love you very much.
We'll always remember
    your gentle touch.

Together – so brief –
    Now worlds apart.
But always together
    Within our hearts.

Stillborn

Born without fanfare.
  Born in the night.
Born with closed eyes
  That never saw light.

Born into this world.
  Born without a cry.
Born without answers
  To the question, "Why?"

No words to express
  The grief that we feel.
A silent prayer spoken
  To comfort and heal.

What can we give them?
  An ear that will hear,
A heart that grieves with them,
  And eyes that shed tears.

Thank you to all the nurses who are supportive to parents through the grief process. Just being there for them helps, and your silence speaks volumes.

Little Voices Still Whisper

Little voices still whisper,
And time after time
I still feel their tears
As their hearts talk to mine.

Then cuddling close
With their breath on my skin
They drift off to sleep
At peace once again.

Secure in the love
and tender embrace,
they rest in the memories
that time can't erase.

I have been blessed by thousands upon thousands of newborns and families who have taught me so much about love, and how to fight for life. I thank them, and our Creator God for such a wonderful gift.

Carry the Lamp

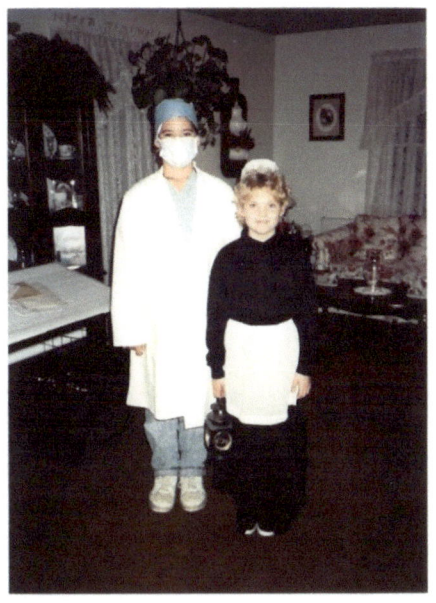

Carry the lamp
Like those gone before.
Care for the sick –
Their health to restore.

Listen to the hearts
That are battered and bruised.
Find a safe haven
For those being abused.

Patch up the wounds,
All the breaks and the broken.
Offer them hope
Through the words that are spoken.

With all that you have
    Help all who have need.
With all that you are
    Uphold the Nurse Creed.

With love and compassion
    Help the sick and the poor.
Yes, carry the lamp
    Till you can't anymore.

Then pass on the light
    So others will see
Hope for the future
    And help for the need.

The Florence Nightingale Pledge

I solemnly pledge myself before God and in the presence of this assembly, to pass my life in purity and to practice my profession faithfully. I will abstain from whatever is deleterious and mischievous, and will not take or knowingly administer any harmful drug. I will do all in my power to maintain and elevate the standard of my profession, and will hold in confidence all personal matters committed to my keeping and all family affairs coming to my knowledge in the practice of my calling. With loyalty will I endeavor to aid the physician in his work, and devote myself to the welfare of those committed to my care.

By Mrs. Lystra E. Gretter 1893

JWH Class of 1974, we made and kept this pledge!

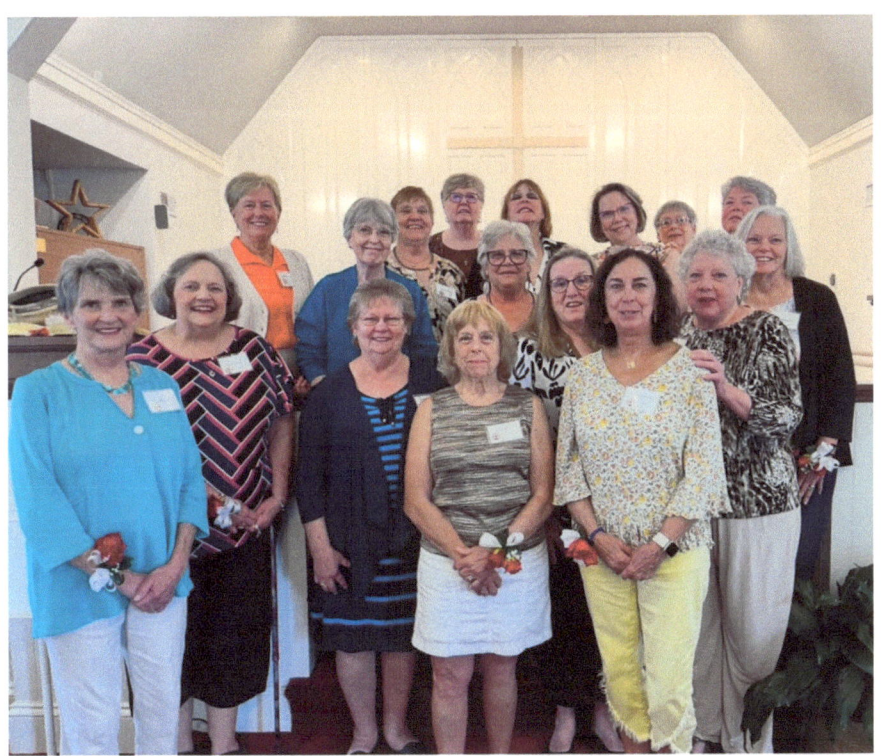

Closure for a Finished Work of Love

How do I say "thank you" to all of the girls?
> You're jewels of the trade – diamonds and pearls.
More precious than metals of silver and gold.
> More valuable than all this – truth be told!

We've weathered the hard times, and came out on top.
> We pressed passed our limits when we wanted to stop.
Exhausted and spent, we'd get up for more.
> Completing our tasks, we'd head for the door.

All of them good days, one way or another
> Whatever our role – friend, sister, or mother.
Together we managed the joys and the strife.
> It's our call, not our job. We celebrate life!

Keep celebrating!

Merry Christmas and Thank You to my family of nurses!

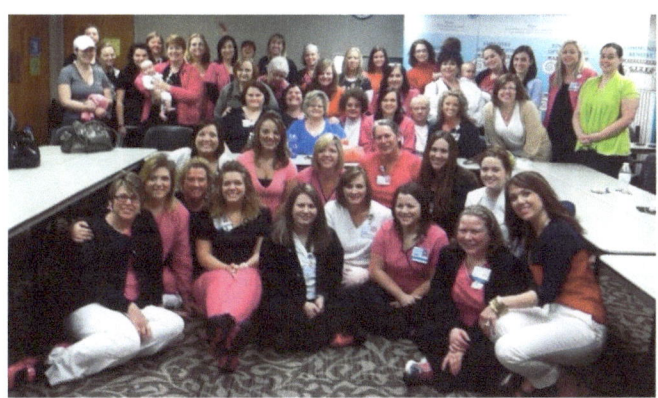

Not Lost, But Found

As I attempt to bring this book to closure, I am submitting a portion of my personal daily journal entry written March 1, 2025:

The little kid inside me feels so lost in this great BIG WORLD! Is that why I climbed trees when I was young, and longed to fly with the birds above it all? Free from the cage, and closer to You? God, I'm trying to express what this feels like – the word that keeps surfacing is "lost".

Then You bring to my mind the line from a poem You gave me for the babies:

"I'm lost in a world of giants, and I'm only hours old..."

You went on to give me the next line for where I am now in life:

> *Where's my Father? Help me find Him!*
> *I'm as desperate as can be!*
> *Then You answer, "I am right here.*
> *Just open your eyes to see."*

❧

I was lost, but now I'm found –
You've never left my side.
When I've needed shelter,
You've been my place to hide.
When I've needed counsel,
You've whispered in my ear.
When I've needed comfort,
You're quick to draw me near.
When I've needed freedom,
You're the One who set me free.
I soar on wings like eagles –
Created by YOU to be ME!

Psalm 118 – God's love never quits!

YES, there's always more!

<u>Thank You</u>

Thank you for taking this walk with me down Memory Lane,
into the Garden Spot of the Hospital.
Each life, like a flower in the Garden of Life, is a precious treasure
sent to bless us in one way or another.
I thank God for the thousands and millions of treasures
He sends to us each and every day all over the world,
and for His plan as the Master Gardner.

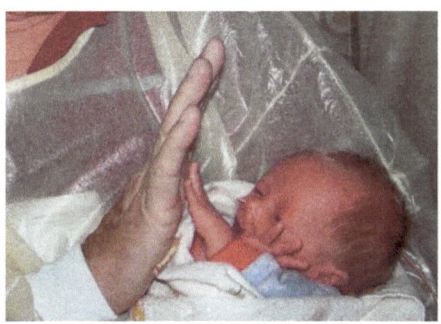

And to each nurse:
May God richly bless you
for the care and comfort, you have provided
to those in need throughout your career.
May He give you an extra measure of grace and mercy,
To go along with your heart of compassion,
in all you do.

Epilogue

As I write this epilogue, I realize that this is not the end of the story. It's an account of a life not yet finished; a journey not yet completed; with a heightened awareness that there's always more to discover!

In some ways I am coming full circle – my early years were filled with dreams of flying like the birds, expressing my thoughts in rhymes, and sketching trees, flowers, birds and bugs. The middle years were consumed with an intense career, and raising children. Now, in my later years, I still dream of flying like the birds, express my thoughts in rhyme and narratives, and art has become a plethora of color on canvas – an overflow of a life full of gratitude. My spirit soars on unseen wings, and I am at peace with myself and the world.

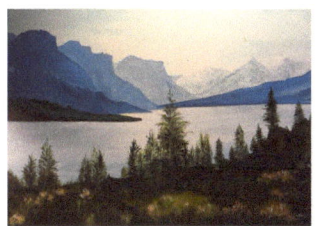

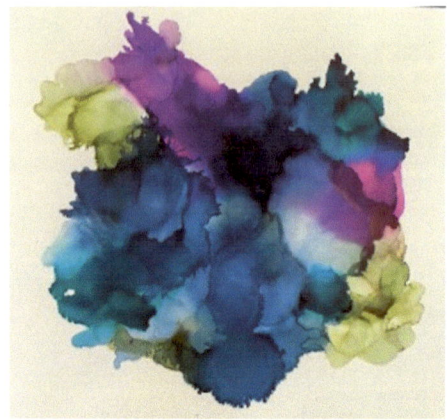

❧

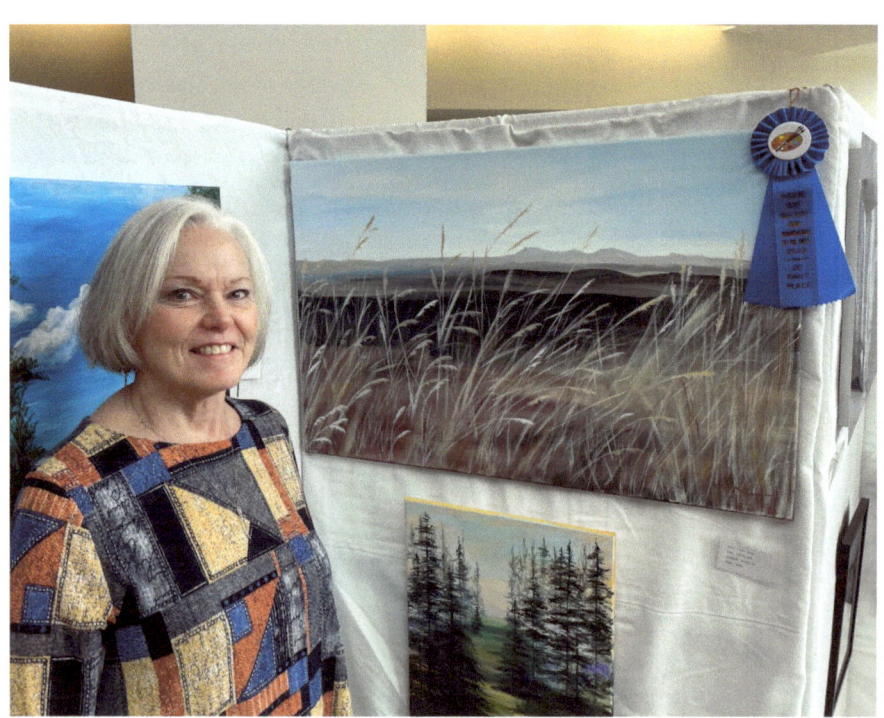

❧

"Our God gives you everything you need,
makes you everything you're to be....
We pray that our God will make you fit
for what He's called you to be,
pray that He'll fill your good ideas
and acts of faith with His own energy
so that it all amounts to something.
If your life honors Jesus, He will honor you.
Grace is behind and through all this,
our God giving Himself freely,
the Master, Jesus Christ, giving Himself freely."

2 Thessalonians 1:2, 11-12 (The Message)

I know this to be true.

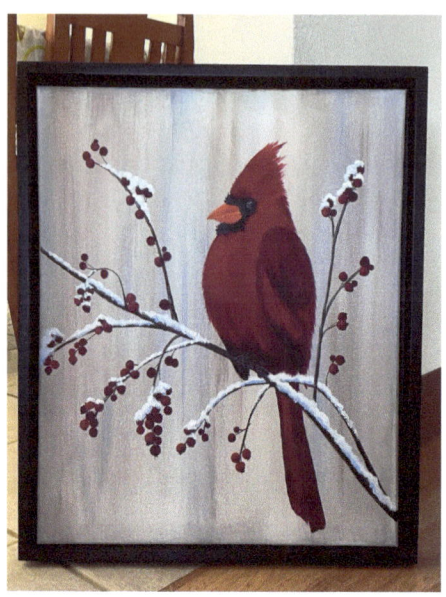

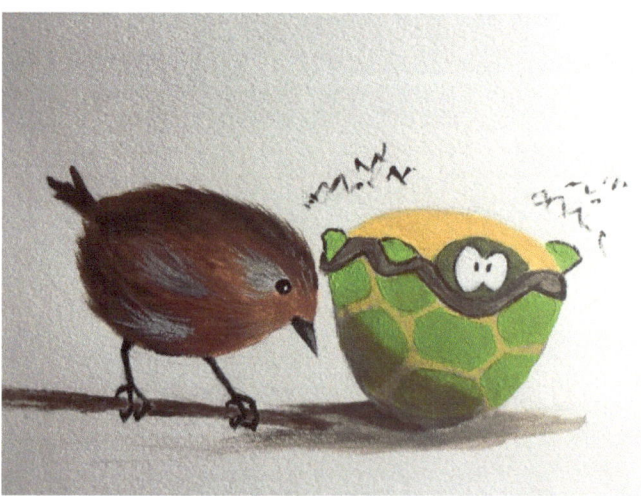

I encourage, and challenge, you to go and search for your true identity. Find out who you really are, and who God created you to be, then step into the reality of your calling. Write it all down. You'll find there's always more.

Go Beyond Me!

About the Author

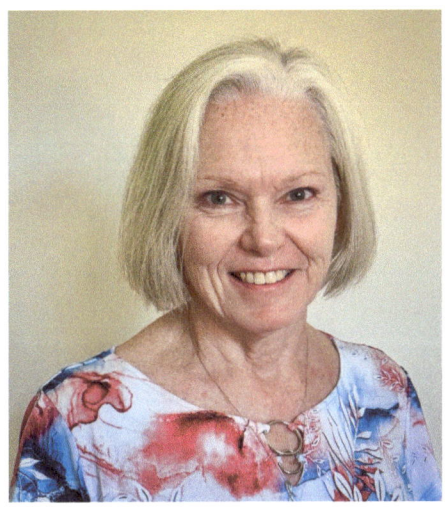

Susan Stiver is a multifaceted diamond in the rough. From her first wall art with red lipstick, to poetry, sketching, a 40-year career in Neonatal Nursing, motherhood, photography, and mixed media art, this lump of coal now has a superabundance of life treasures to expound upon in narrative form. Her passion is to communicate the heart of God through her writing and art, expressing God's love and desire for each individual to know and be known by Him.

For this lifetime writer, rhyme has been a creative and emotional outlet – a means to convey thoughts, questions, and muses that inspire and encourage others. Her poetry is a dance with words, and heart-whispers scribed on paper with ink.

The world is so full of God-wonders; little miracles are born every day. This book is a tribute to those little miracles, their families, and to the care providers.

Other Books

He Loves You to Pieces

A Heart Stirred for Fellowship
Co-authored with her husband
Don Stiver

A Walk in the Garden
Go Beyond Me
Book One

The Ebb and Flow of Life and Family
Go Beyond Me
Book Two

Contact the Author
Susanstiver212@gmail.com

www.ingramcontent.com/pod-product-compliance
Lightning Source LLC
Chambersburg PA
CBHW040845120626
46547CB00001B/31